The Exploitation of Desire: Women's Experiences with In Vitro Fertilisation

ABOUT THE AUTHOR

Renate D. Klein has a biology degree from Zurich University and degrees in Women's Studies from the University of California, Berkeley and London University. She is co-editor with Rita Arditti and Shelley Minden of *Test-Tube Women: What Future for Motherhood?* (1984) and co-author with Gena Corea et al. of *Man–Made Women* (1985). She is a founding member of the Feminist International Network of Resistance to Reproductive and Genetic Engineering (FINRRAGE) and an editor of *Reproductive and Genetic Engineering: Journal of International Feminist Analysis.* Her book *Infertility: Women Speak out about Their Experiences Of Reproductive Medicine* will appear in 1989 (Pandora Press, London/ Allen & Unwin, Sydney). She is currently a Research Fellow at Deakin University.

★

Cover Design — Concrete Poem by thalia —
Treatments Abnormal Patience

Concrete poetry is a play on a letter or word to give you a visual effect. Here the poet becomes printer, for it deals expressly with the effects of writing.

Language has a visual contact.

★

ACKNOWLEDGEMENTS

I gratefully acknowledge the support of the Australian Federation of University Women who awarded me the 1986–87 Georgina Sweet Fellowship which enabled me to pursue the initial research for this project. I also thank the Women's Studies Programme, School of Humanities, and Deakin University for appointing me as their Post-Doctoral Research Fellow from 1987–89.

THE EXPLOITATION OF A DESIRE

— RENATE KLEIN —

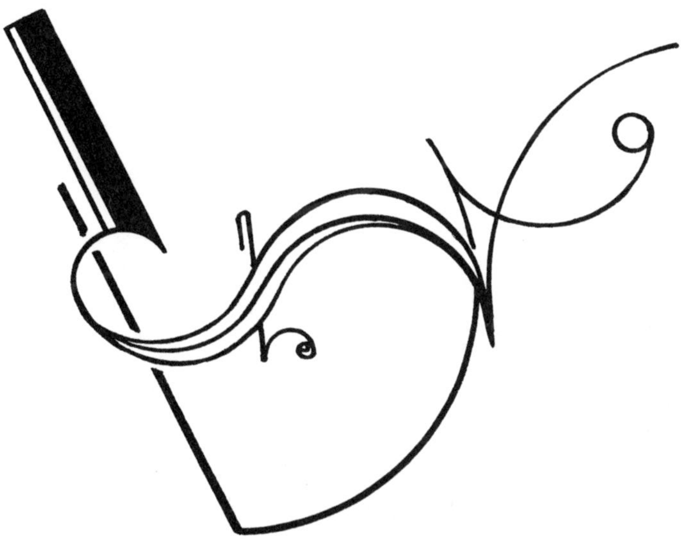

TREATMENTS

ABNORMAL

PATIENCE

Published by Women's Studies Summer Institute
Distributed by Deakin University Press, Geelong, Victoria 3217, Australia

Typeset in Goudy 11 on 12 by
Dead Set, Fitzroy, Victoria 3065
Printed in Australia by
Ellikon Printers, Fitzroy, Victoria 3065

National Library of Australia
Cataloguing-in-Publication

Klein, R. D., 1945–
The exploitation of a desire : women's experiences with in vitro fertilisation.
ISBN 0 7300 0287 X
Bibliography.

1. Fertilisation in vitro, Human. 2. Human reproduction — Social aspects. 3. Women — Health and hygiene. I. Deakin University Women's Studies Summer Institute

618.1'78

CONTENTS

For all the women
who say NO *to*
reproductive technology.

PREFACE

In the social debate surrounding the development of the new reproductive technologies one group has been notable by their silence: the thousands of women who have suffered the negative efforts of reproductive technology programmes internationally. At last, in this exploratory survey, Renate Klein has enabled a group of Australian women to give voice to their experiences.

I am delighted, as Director of the Deakin University Women's Studies Summer Institute, to be able to publish this work which Dr Klein has carried out in her capacity as Post-Doctoral Research Fellow in Women's Studies in the School of Humanities. The report gives us glimpses into the lives of women as we see close-up, and for the first time, how women look back on the story of infertility in their lives, on the decisions with which they grappled while on IVF programmes and on how their wishes and experiences were ignored. We also learn how they experience themselves as 'guinea pigs' within the power play of technodocs. The pain, both physical and emotional, comes through these voices and women show the considerable strength that is required to deal with the many conflicts and contradictions within a society that has no regard for women without children.

We can only appreciate the courage of the women who speak up in this study. We can only thank Renate Klein for breaking their silence. We can only hope that reading this report will encourage other women to speak out and break the misleading myths generated about these experimental technologies. And we can work to make sure that the voices in this report will be heard in various government committee sittings where only users who advocate continuation of these technologies have so far been heard. Perhaps then, these dangerous, expensive and failed technologies will be abandoned by government and community alike.

Dr Robyn Rowland
Melbourne, January 1989

INTRODUCTION

Since the birth of the first child conceived *in vitro* (in the glass) outside a woman's body in 1978 — Louise Brown in England — the 'test-tube baby method' has been a highly sought-after media topic internationally.

Most frequently *in vitro* fertilisation (IVF) is hailed as a benevolent technological revolution that provides infertile couples with their 'last chance' to have their deeply wished for biological child. The message we get is one of benevolent *progress*; of dedicated scientists and doctors working hard to alleviate the pain of involuntary childlessness. And of science conquering the possibly last frontier: taking control of procreation where nature 'fails'.[1] By focusing on the few hours that it takes for the egg cell and sperm to fertilise in the laboratory dish and divide into an 4–8 cell embryo which is then inserted into the woman's womb — and highlighting this part of the experience of the becoming of a new human being by calling the children 'test-tube' or 'IVF' babies, human reproduction has been taken out of the realm of 'the private' — that is the woman's body — and instead entered into 'the public': the controlled environment of laboratories and hospitals.

And yet the fact remains that it continues to be *women* who are the main actors in this modern reproduction drama; at least till the perfection of the artificial womb and the maturation of immature eggs *in vitro* — two 'hot' research topics currently investigated by the international scientific research community.[2] It is *women* who provide the mature egg cells, and it is *women* who have the inserted foetus/embryo develop as part of their own bodies for the nine months' pregnancy period. In fact, in those rare instances when IVF works, it is women (without or with a partner) and not the 'fathers' from the laboratory who will be the mothers of their child(ren) for life.

What do these women feel, think and experience in their journey from wishing for a biological child to encountering difficulties conceiving and eventually undergoing IVF? How do the technological interventions, from taking fertility drugs for egg maturation, to having egg cells removed and embryos inserted, influence their lives? Their physical and emotional well-being? Their sense of Self? And how do those for whom it does not work feel — *the average 90–95 women out of 100* who quit IVF without a child?[3]

Reviewing the international literature — scientific and popular alike — these are questions that are *not* asked. With the exception of a growing body of writings by concerned feminists[4] of which this work is part, women in IVF are invisible. Or, if they are mentioned at all, it is as 'uterine environments', as 'the best incubators God provides', as factories of 'a good egg crop' — not as *whole* people. Even when criticism about IVF is voiced it is either economic in nature ('the cost-benefit ratio is unsatisfactory') or *foetalist*, that is, it is concerned with questions about the beginning of life and the status of the embryo rather than *feminist*: focusing on the impact of these technologies on *women's* lives.[5] Lacking, also, is the debate that the development of reproductive technology on human beings must be seen as part of the whole development of biotechnology and specifically genetic engineering of plants, animals and human beings.[6] And it is not discussed that to have women available as 'egg providers' — of eggs that can be manufactured into embryos in the laboratory — is the indispensable condition for embryo experimentation (Rowland, 1987): Experimentation which in turn enables the manipulation of genes and which can lead to further social control of who is 'worthy' to reproduce and who is not — the old eugenics in a new technological guise.[7]

The obvious paradox, that women are the main actors in IVF and, in theory, hold a considerable amount of power, but, at the same time, are being rendered invisible and their desire for a child is exploited — would be sufficient justification for an investigation of the impact of these technologies on women's lives. Are they in control of these procedures which, supposedly, were invented 'for their own good' (Ehrenreich and English, 1978)? If there are problems, what can be done about them? What — and who — ensures that these technologies are really in women's best interests? And what does 'women's best interests' mean in a patriarchal world in which a 'proper' woman continues to be equated with a woman with child; a world that continues to be male-dominated, in which women — 52 per cent of the world's population — are the poor, sick, illiterate, own only one percent of the world's resources and earn only ten percent while doing two thirds of the work (United Nations Statistics, 1980). What do terms like 'choice' and 'procreative liberty' mean used by the promoters of these technologies when they talk of women 'voluntarily' entering IVF programmes in Western countries while they decide that single, lesbian, and poor women are 'unsuitable' candidates; whereas, by contrast, the majority of women in so-called Third World countries are forced into childlessness via sterilisation or harmful contraceptives?[8]

Yet there was another reason that prompted me to undertake this exploratory survey. IVF is not without danger. Firstly, in order to 'harvest' the egg cells, the most frequently employed surgical invasion which requires anaesthesia — laparoscopy — may prove fatal. Indeed, there is proof that at least eleven women have died while on IVF programmes in Israel, France, Germany, Martinique (Corea, personal communication, 1988), Brazil (Gomez Dos Reis, 1987) and Perth, Australia (1987 and 1988). Secondly, disturbing evidence is accumulating that the hormones administered to stimulate the growth of egg follicles can lead not only to superovulation (the maturation of more than one ripe egg) but also to *hyper*stimulation. This hyperstimulation in turn may produce ovarian cysts and there are a number of reported cases of the promotion of cancer. In one particularly gruesome case in England, cancerous cells spread from both ovaries to appendix, uterus and bladder (Carter and Joyce, 1987: 126–128) all of which had to be removed in order to save the woman's life. It thus appears that the administration of what French gynaecologist, Dr Anne Cabau, calls 'explosive cocktails' (1986:3), that is, the application of a mixture of hormones to stimulate the growth of egg follicles, may indeed endanger the lives of *healthy* women. Also, a time-bomb may be ticking in the prescription of Clomiphene citrate — frequently sold as Clomid, a fertility drug used internationally in both 'conventional' infertility treatments as well as IVF. It bears a very close structural similarity to DES (Diethystilbestrol), a drug prescribed, from the 1940s to the 1970s, to millions of pregnant women supposedly prone to miscarriage which resulted in 3–5 million daughters and sons with fertility problems, and, in the case of the daughters, increased incidence of cancer of the vagina and the cervix as well as increased rates of breast cancers for the mothers.[9] The risk is that in 20 years' time mothers who were given these 'IVF cocktails' may suffer serious ill health, if not death, caused by cancer, and that children born of such treatments may suffer fates similar to DES offspring (see Klein/Rowland, 1988).

The question I pursued in my research was, does a woman contemplating IVF know about the possibility of such dangers? Put differently, in addition to investigating the impact of IVF on women's lives in general. I was concerned with finding out whether the clinics offered information to the women prior to their taking these hormones as to the potential short and long-term 'side' effects. Are they informed about what hormonal 'mixtures' they are given? And above all, is it made clear to them that — contrary to media reporting — IVF remains an *experimental* procedure in which, because every woman reacts differently, there is no such thing as a 'standard' hormonal dose but only the trial and error method, which may easily lead to hyperstimulation and the formation of cysts.

Furthermore, I wanted to know what women who contemplate IVF are told about its success rate. Is there an attempt to tell them the *real* success rates, that is the percentage of *live* babies compared with all the women who began IVF; or, as Gena Corea and Susan Ince (1987) have shown of US clinics, were they deluded with massaged success rates which counted as successes: chemical pregnancies, tubal pregnancies, and spontaneous abortions (though none will yield a live child). Corea and Ince found that clinics did *not* count women who are eliminated from the programme before the laparoscopic egg retrieval stage; screening or diagnostic laparoscopies that do *not* yield a pregnancy; and laparoscopic egg retrievals that do not result in any embryo transfer' (p.135). As an IVF expert himself put it: 'It's too easy to fudge results' (Alan de Cherney of Yale University in Corea and Ince, 1987:135). I wanted to know what the practice of Australian doctors is?

In sum, my research was motivated by the growing concern of feminists worldwide that IVF is *not* in women's best interests, that it is a failed technology and that it might in fact be dangerous for women to undergo an IVF procedure. This exploratory survey is a first attempt to find women who have actually undergone IVF and who will speak for themselves about their experiences.

Methodology

It was important for me to ensure that the women who spoke out about their IVF experiences would do so unconstrained by outside forces, such as personnel from an IVF programme. As I will discuss in the last chapter (Discussion), many women, although very sceptical about the technologies and critical of practitioners, for a variety of reasons do not want to speak out publicly against IVF. It also seemed ethically advisable to restrict my investigation to women who had stopped participating in the IVF programme.[10]

For these reasons, in December 1986 I placed advertisements in two major newspapers in Melbourne (*The Age*, *The Herald*),[11] asking women who had undergone IVF to participate in a survey about IVF. I guaranteed full anonymity and explained that participation would include filling in a questionnaire with the possibility of taking part in a follow-up interview. I immediately received fifteen requests for questionnaires and within the next month another seven queries. Interviews with me in *The Sun* and *The Geelong Advertiser* (February 1987), brought a furthther ten requests from women willing to participate and by the end of May 1987, I had sent out a total of forty-three questionnaires, forty of which were completed and returned (93%).[12]

Without exception, the women indicated their names, addresses and phone numbers and stated their willingness to participate in a follow-up interview. In addition, a good third mentioned at the end that it had been important for them — though as many said painful — to complete this questionnaire and to know that someone was concerned about them and their experiences (see Findings for further comments on these statements).

By the end of May 1987 I had undertaken twenty-five follow-up interviews. In addition, after the above mentioned interviews with me in the two newspapers as well as two talks I gave at Melbourne University (March) and the Victorian chapter of the Australian Federation of University Women (April), I also was contacted by over twenty women who shared their own or a friend's experience with me and who were willing to provide further information. Two-thirds had been on IVF programmes in the Melbourne area, the rest came from South Australia, Western Australia and the ACT.

As this work is part of an international research project to assess the experiences of women with conventional infertility treatment, IVF and surrogacy (to be published in an anthology, 1989[13]) constant interaction with my contributors was invaluable as they helped place my research within the context of the international movement of feminists concerned with the impact of these technologies on women's lives.[14] Last but not least, this research project profited greatly from discussions with my Australian colleagues and FINRRAGE members Robyn Rowland, Christine Ewing, Sarah Ferber, Christine Crowe, Lariane Fonseca, Jocelynne Scutt, Ditta Bartels and US researchers Gena Corea and Janice Raymond[15]

The questionnaire was long and time-consuming to complete. It consisted of 186 questions in seven Sections: A Personal Data; B Infertility; C Treatment(s) before IVF; D Commencing IVF; E The IVF Procedure; F Problems; G The Time After IVF. Some of the questions were quick 'yes/no' answers, others asked specifically about details of the IVF procedures (e.g. number of attempts, number of eggs recovered, financial cost, etc.), but the main emphasis was on open-ended questions. In agreement with other feminist researchers (e.g. Du Bois, Mies, and Reinharz in Bowles and Duelli Klein, 1983) the use of quantitative research methodology appears problematic to me. For that reason, I mentioned in the covering letter I sent with the questionnaire that I did *not* plan to evaluate the answers statistically, but that I intended to use them as the starting point for the follow-up interviews.

As in the prior surveys I have conducted (Duelli Klein 1980, 1986), my scepticism about the value of questionnaires was confirmed: it is usually only in an in-depth interview, after establishing a degree of personal interaction between interviewee and interviewer, that the words put on paper begin to be meaningful, i.e. when linked with other pieces of information they shed some light on the full range of the participant's experiences (see also Oakley, 1981). In many cases it was also obvious that to be able to talk about the IVF experience and to see a person in the flesh who was interested in her experience, made the woman say much more radical things than she previously had put on the page. In fact, in many cases, a written statement took on a totally different meaning when we discussed it.

It is important in this context to state that I said from the beginning (already in the covering letter, restating it in the interview) that I was a critic of IVF and worried that it was *not* in women's best interests. Contrary to my apprehension that some women may become hostile or be annoyed by this, they all — without exception — respected my stance. In fact, about two-thirds of them agreed that one could certainly see problems with IVF, even if they themselves had chosen to ignore them (or were not aware of them at the time; see Findings for further details) and were not as strongly opposed to it as me.

The point I wish to make here is that all the completed questionnaires and especially the interviews show the participants in my survey as articulate and reflective women whose desire for a child had led them to embark on a problematic enterprise which not only proved to be very difficult, but also unsuccessful. It appears, however, that precisely by wanting to take part in my study, they demonstrate that they have learnt to live with this unsuccessful result and coped with the fact that their/their partner's wish for a(nother) child remained unfulfilled. Many, in fact, have put the past behind them and reflect on their IVF experience as a part of that past that is over and done with.[16]

Finally then, before I turn to the women's experiences, I would like to discuss the validity of this exploratory survey. The following pages reveal a lot of pain, false expectations, disappointment and anger. Critics might say that my study does not encompass women who have been content with their IVF experience (despite the fact that it was not successful). To them, want to respond forcefully that I believe the reverse is true: that there is a bias in my study towards women who felt they *could* cope with their IVF experience, who *were* emotionally capable of writing and talking about it. Almost without exception they are well-educated and middle class. Almost without exception they had strong support from their husbands. This finding does counter other, more anecdotal stories about women from IVF programmes whose partner first pushed them into the programme and then reacted so badly when it did not work that their marriage broke up with the result that they were totally destroyed by the experience. In fact, we know of a number of suicides and of women who became alcoholics in order to forget the experience of the continuous pain of involuntary childlessness exacerbated by repeated IVF attempts.

In other words, I believe that the often harsh words that will follow reveal only the tip of the iceberg of what women have to go through in their IVF experience. It is my contention that those whose lives were wrecked by the trauma of being 'living laboratories' (Rowland, 1984:364) in the hands of some particularly ruthless, success-orientated and misogynist doctors and scientists did *not* reply to the advertisement in the paper. From some of the stories I have heard it appears that they may be too 'broken by patriarchy'[17] even to be able to try and work through what happened to them. Because there are no services provided for the overwhelming majority of women for whom IVF does not work, there is no place for them to go: they are thrown by the wayside and left to their own devices. If, in the meantime, their marriage has broken up and they feel responsible for that too (as well as feeling 'failures' about IVF) they are much worse off than before they embarked on IVF. This is one of the many facts about the IVF procedure which I think are scandalous and I will return to it in the final chapter (Discussion). This is why I have come to believe, through hearing the women's stories about their experiences, that IVF represents *a new form of violence against women: a violation of women's human dignity*. And this is why I think IVF —a failed technology — must be stopped.[18]

FINDINGS

Personal Data

Twenty women — half of the participants in my study — were between 30 and 35 years old, three were under 20 and five over 40. Twelve were between 35 and 40 years old. Their partners were somewhat older: twelve over 40, eleven between 35 and 40, fifteen between 30 and 35, and two under 30. With the exception of two women who were in *de facto* relationships, all were married at the time(s) when they were on the IVF programme: sixteen women had been in the relationship for 5–10 years, fourteen for over 10 years and eight for under 5 years. Two of the women did not respond to this question. At the time of my survey, this had changed very little: only one woman said she was single, the others had remained in the same type of relationship with the same partners. Thirty women described their relationships as 'generally happy', eight as 'mixed' and two as 'very happy'. None ticked the category 'generally unhappy'. (See also the section below, Infertility, for further comments on and its influence on the nature of women's relationships.)

More than half of the women (twenty-three) listed 'Protestant' as their religious affiliation, eleven stated 'nil', four cited 'Roman Catholic' and two 'Eastern'. Twenty-four described their cultural background as Australian, ten as British, four as European and two as New Zealanders. Nineteen said their highest level of education was 'secondary' and thirteen said 'tertiary' (six TAFE, 7 degrees); six listed 'low secondary' and two did not respond to the question. Their partners' highest levels of education were tertiary degree (11), secondary (19), and low secondary (6). Four did not respond to the question.

With regard to occupation, a relatively large number of the women in my sample — seventeen — were nurses (SRN and SEN). Four others were teachers; seven listed 'home duties', five 'clerical', three 'cook', and four 'other' as their occupation. Their partners' occupations were professional (11), other white collar (9), trade (6), other blue collar (11). Three did not respond to the question. Thirty-three described their income as medium at the time of IVF, five as 'high' and two as 'low'. While the majority of women (thirty-five) were in paid employment before IVF, ten gave up work, four went part-time and two took long-service leave while on IVF. At the time of my study only twenty-six were employed — which is a marked drop from thirty-five prior to IVF.

With regard to the time spent on the IVF programme, for a large number of women, it was 2 years (19), for ten 1 year, for seven 3 years and for four 4 years. During this time, they said they spent between 1 and 3 months each year on the programme. As to the total number of IVF attempts, nineteen women underwent three attempts, eleven had two, four had five attempts. Three women tried only once, while three others tried IVF eight times. The IVF procedure(s) cost thirteen women between $3,000 and $4,000, seven between $5,000 and $6,000, five over $6,000 and three under $2,000. (The other women could not remember.) The majority said they were refunded roughly half of the cost.

Infertility

There is no doubt that infertility can be a shattering experience. As one woman put it:

> *I felt emotionally distraught, worthless, extremely upset, and angry. It was bitter disappointment, social rejection — a feeling of being incomplete.*

Half the women in my study (n = 40), that is 20, ranked infertility as 'a very upsetting experience'. Twelve others said that it was 'the worst experience that ever happened to me', while eight felt that it was 'disappointing but so were other things that did not work in my life'. Of the women in my study, twenty-seven were the infertile part in their relationship — five due to a tubal ligation. In eight cases no reason for the infertility could be found (idiopathic infertility), while in five cases the infertility had been diagnosed as her partner's problem. It should be mentioned that seven women had children (2–5) from a previous relationship and three had a child from the present partner *before* the fertility problem. Five men, too, had children (1–2) from previous relationships. Also, in six cases the couple had a child *after* unsuccessful IVF (that is their fertility problem was overcome 'naturally'). Eleven had adopted a child and seven were still in the process of adoption.

For sixteen women it was 3–5 years since they had found out about the infertility, for fifteen 6–9 years and seven over 10 years. Two did not respond to the question. In those cases in which the nature of the infertility had been diagnosed, it was damaged or blocked fallopian tubes (14) — this includes the five women with tubal ligations, endometriosis (6), presence of antibodies (3), hostile mucus (2), adhesions (1), inflamed appendix (1), and low/no sperm count (5). Two did not respond to the question.

As to the *cause(s)* of the fertility problem, twelve women said that they were told it was *not known*, ten said they were *not told*, six mentioned pelvic inflammatory disease (PID), six others put 'infection'. Three of the PID and three of the 'infection' group put infertility down to problems from an IUD. Two other women were told it was due to a 'bad' abortion, one to an appendix operation. One put 'age' and two did not respond to the question.

Once the women had undertaken steps to find out why they did not get pregnant and saw a doctor, the majority of them — thirty-one — only told family and close friends about the problem. Four others included 'colleagues'. Only five women said that they talked to anyone who said, 'Why no baby?' or would listen.

What became very clear from the women's responses is the enormous stigma attached to infertility. Not being able to have one's own biological children for many people amounts to suffering from a disease. As one woman put it:

> *Our families — and particularly my in-laws — were shocked and, as they told me, disappointed not to have grandchildren. Since the day I told them they've treated me very condescendingly . . . with a mixture of pity and contempt: somewhere along the lines that I now was a sick person who could not be taken seriously.*

Another woman remembers a rather traumatic evening:

> *After the gynaecologist had spoken the verdict "blocked tubes", I went straight to a birthday party for one of my best friends. I couldn't contain myself and broke the news to everyone. But I got quite annoyed with the responses. I'm sure they meant well but within minutes I was swamped with advice that ranged from 'See a herbalist' to "try IVF" and from "cold baths" to "relax". I got really angry when one of Alan's friends offered to "fill in" — so that I could be shown how 'one really makes babies'. It was the first and last time I mentioned the infertility in public.*

It is particularly evident that many people simply do not want to accept the possibility that some people who cannot have children can nevertheless live happy lives after they have accepted the fertility problem and grieved over the desire for a child that was not to be. This stigmatisation sets the scene for many people's long and painful journey from one infertility treatment to another: in today's world more and more frequently culminating in IVF. As one woman remembers:

There's one lady at work who's got three kids and she just won't have the infertility. She said, "Look, I've got a friend who had her first baby at 40, and you've still got 4 years to go, and you know, you're not to give up."
And I said, "Yes, but I'm sick of it, you know, it's been 13 years and I've had enough."
"No," she said, "you can't give up. Not yet!"

Because having children is still the norm to which Australian society[19] at large expects a 'proper' woman to aspire, many involuntary childless women feel like outcasts. The following comment stands for many similar sentiments:

Increasingly, I felt displaced at family events. Everyone had children but us. And although I'd just been promoted I know Mum's eyes would have lighted up much more if I had announced "I'm pregnant".

As many as twenty women mentioned during the interviews that they had lost a lot of friends, families who found them 'odd' or envied them 'for our overseas trip and a nice house — things I would have quickly given up for a baby.' The same women also remarked that they longed for friends *without* children — especially women friends — and how difficult it was to find them.

Because society expects women to have children, people with an infertility problem are endlessly encouraged to 'try once more'. The possibility to talk about difficulties of involuntary childlessness and to grieve in public, so to speak, in order to start on a new phase in life, does not exist. There is also a deeply entrenched sexist attitude that infertility must be the *woman's* problem. One woman who knew, through painful tests, that she had fully functioning ovaries and tubes but whose husband's sperm had low motility remembers that her mother-in-law did not want to know anything about her son being infertile 'almost as if it was an insult to *her*'. Another woman said:

> *Eventually I told more and more people that it was Norm's problem because everybody assumed it was my fault and I felt very pressured by their patronising approach to me.*

Due to such pressure, many women internalise the infertility problem. Despite the fact that a substantial number of women in my study were either not told what caused the infertility (10) or were told that it was not known (12) or became infertile after an infection/PID (6) — often from IUDs — thirty women said that they have felt guilty about the infertility. This includes even women from the group with idiopathic infertility and those who did not know the cause(s):

> *Although no definite reason had been given for our infertility I did feel guilty and I feel responsible for the problem mainly because my first husband had remarried and has a child by his second wife.*

Others explained their guilt feelings in the following ways:

> *I felt I had deprived my husband of the chance of being a parent.*

> *Had I left it too late? Was it taking the pill too long? Why me?*

> *Especially as in my twenties I had several sex partners I feel I may have stuffed up my reproductive system through contracting PID.*

> *I felt guilty because I was involuntarily withholding something that had become very important to him. Also I felt guilt about an abortion at 16.*

From the five men who had been diagnosed as having the fertility problem, only one said he felt guilty. One other woman commented on this question:

> *When our first results proved only that there was a problem with my husband he felt guilty, but when the second lot of tests proved that there were problems on both sides, the situation was entirely different.*

'Guilt', 'stigma' — and woman blaming — mix in the case of PID. As one woman put it:

Pelvic inflammatory disease carries a certain stigma much like venereal diseases. As my husband is a doctor I was really embarrassed that his colleagues might think that his wife had "slept around".

From all these remarks it is not surprising to learn that as many as twelve women — almost one-third of the women in my study (n = 40) — suggested divorce to their partners (in contrast, only three men brought up the possibility of divorce). One woman said:

It got to the point where each time we were arguing or having a fight or something I tell him to go and find himself a fertile woman.

As many as thirty-two women said that the infertility took a heavy toll on their relationship. Twelve felt that in the end the infertility problem had strengthened their relationship, but that, when undergoing the various treatments, it had been very stressful. One woman summarises these reflections succinctly:

In the end it has brought us closer together in communicating with each other. Adversely, it has affected our sexual relations as the futility of trying to become pregnant foreshadows the pleasurable aspects of sex.

Ten women saw the influence to be more negative than positive:

It caused a lot of tension; we faced enormous emotional problems and had to decide if we would remain together as a couple.

Four others, however, said that in the end their relationship had gained from the many years of struggling with infertility (including IVF). As one woman put it:

I doubt that anything could come between us now. Especially when we were on the [IVF] programme we had no help as to how it would affect us and how our emotions would go up and down. We had to cope with all our emotional problems and we did.

And another woman said:

It caused a lot of tension and put a different angle on our life. We now want different things out of life. One of the reasons I married him was because he'd make a good father.

In sum, then, many women experience infertility as a serious life crisis. Because of society's rarely challenged assumptions that having children is the 'normal' thing to do for a mature woman — thus implicitly stigmatising *her* irrespective of the nature of the fertility problem — many women's self-esteem and well being are seriously affected by infertility. It is important to note that often their whole sense of self becomes shaky; in other words that they experience 'a feeling of being displaced', 'of not belonging'. Or, as one woman said: 'I felt anger, despair, hurt, was upset and thought it was so unfair. It was like my whole world had fallen apart and I was floundering with no future.'

It is crucial to recognise such overwhelming and all-encompassing emotions that many women experience once the dreaded verdict 'infertility' has been pronounced. I believe it shows that women who are de-stabilised at the very core of their sense of self by this event — 'I felt a failure to myself', as one said — can only rarely be helped by the 'technological fixes' that conventional infertility treatments — but in particular IVF — offer. Only few of them — if any — see themselves as the 'defective machines' that need to be fixed up (like a car) which is the very *basis* of reproductive medicine ('old' and 'new' version). For many, the infertility triggers complex reactions, for instance the regret about not being able to experience the loving and spoiling of a very special and precious human being — especially when still helpless and dependent on such care and responsibility. 'Social rejection' loomed large and frequently, as did the sheer helplessness they felt when confronted with the fact that something they hid always taken for granted — a child of their own — seemed all of a sudden denied for life.[20]

Because I believe that many of the women in my study experienced the infertility in this 'holistic' way, it does not seem very surprising that a substantial number of them tried to deal with this life crisis in a radical way. Twenty-six women mentioned that they did contemplate a different road than the one they ended up taking. Put differently, rather than beginning the endless and traumatic journey of infertility treatments, these women said they would have gone for adoption at the time the infertility was diagnosed. Eight women also commented that life without biological children seemed a possibility and mentioned the many possibilities of 'social mothering'. With regard to adoption, some were told they were too old (three), others were rejected (three) and others *did* adopt after IVF (eleven) or are still on the waiting list (seven). But in sixteen cases, it had been the *husband* who was against adoption or a 'child-free life' — more than a third in my study — a strong force in pushing women to seek a medical solution in addition to the above mentioned pressures exercised by society at large. And once on the medical treadmill of the treatment — as we have already seen — it is almost impossible to stop.

Treatments Before IVF

It is important to realise that until recently[21] most women beginning IVF brought with them a long, painful and disappointing history of failed medical interventions — 'years and years of pre-IVF horror stories' as one woman said — sometimes including artificial insemination. The following two women are not alone with their experiences:

> *Firstly, I followed graphs to show ovulation, restricting intercourse to fertile times; then referral to gyno. First gyno, again, graphs about fertile times, then tubular X-rays show blockage. Second gyno; laparoscopy, found endometriosis, six months Danocrin which cleared endometriosis. Clomid for six months and ultrascan to see whether I was ovulating, monthly blood tests to check ovulation and planning intercourse at peak, after intercourse mucus tests and when all that failed AI — artificial insemination by husband.*

> *First mucus tests on me; second mucus plus sperm tests; third laparoscopy; fourth salpingogram — dreadful. Tubal surgery — dreadful. Microsurgery, more sperm and more mucus tests with donor controls. Naturopath and finally IVF.*

Their partners — at wost — had to have a sperm test done and this often only *after* the women had already undergone a number of painful tests to establish their (in)fertility.

Artificial insemination was considered by fifteen couples (for fourteen it was not applicable because of blocked or no tubes). Only six, however, attempted it and were without success. One woman commented that her husband thought it to be more stressful than IVF. One of the women whose partner was infertile commented that

> *We rejected AID because my husband wanted his own biological children.*

Gamete intrafallopian transfer (GIFT) was attempted by ten women without success.

In sum, treatments before IVF are mostly long and painful, interfere with work and often lead to ill health. Four women in my study had ovarian cysts developing from the prolonged hyperstimulation with hormones and had to have them removed via laparotomy. In one case, carcinoma was suspected. Tubal surgery almost unavoidably brought with it antibiotics so the women's bodies — in the quest to repair 'defective' parts — were thrown off natural balance. Importantly, even before they began IVF, the women already had a long history of 'failure': the many treatments they undertook did not bring them the child they wished for. Or, if indeed a pregnancy began, it ended in a miscarriage or was diagnosed as multiple and/or ectopic. Notwithstanding this long history of 'not expecting it to work', the unsuccessful experience of IVF — as discussed in the next sections — seems to be incomparably worse — 'devastating' as many women called it — a phenomenon that needs explanation.

Commencing IVF

Thirty-two women (n = 40) had been told by their gynaecologists about IVF. An equal number (though not all the same women) had read the IVF 'success-stories' in the newspapers and glossy magazines. Other sources frequently cited were TV (twenty-nine) and radio (13),[22] while 'colleagues at work', 'female friends', 'parents' and 'siblings' were only rarely mentioned.

The first impressions of IVF were overwhelmingly positive. As one woman put it:

> *I remember thinking it was a sure thing and that participation would be no trouble.*

Another remembered:

It seemed like a promise, a new technology for women. But it is not.

Memory about success rates was poor but one woman spoke for many when she said, 'I assumed every person succeeded — ha ha ha.'

A few, however, remembered exact figures that ranged from 50% to 30–40% to 20%. Only one woman said she heard 5% and another between 12% and 17%.

Asked about their initial reaction about trying for themselves, 'It was one of excitement, hope and great expectation' for many (29). One woman clearly remembered her initial feelings:

I was delighted, my husband thrilled; we felt very privileged, optimistic, keen to participate. Although we knew it was a chance factor we thought it would be helpful to have positive thoughts. Psychologically it might help to have them anyway. We were very happy. We knew it was perhaps a way to achieve our baby. We clung to any hope as we knew we were getting older. It gave us new hope.

Only a few women said they felt 'uneasy' and 'apprehensive' from the beginning; many felt 'It was the last opportunity open to us' (twenty-two) or:

A chance was better than none; at least we could say that we'd tried the latest technology.

'Absolutely sure' that the procedure would work were only six women, while the majority (twenty-eight) said they had some doubts but hoped for the best. Four women commented that they never really did believe that IVF would work for them. (In this question their partners' responses were almost identical.)

Thirty-five women, however, did see problems with IVF: for thirty it was 'the worry that IVF might not work', for twenty-five 'the financial costs involved' (multiple checking of answers was possible). Twenty-five women also ticked 'the possibility that you might not be able to cope with the emotional stress while on the programme'. Only six women envisaged 'the possibility that the IVF procedure might harm your body', and even fewer — four — had fears that something could be wrong with a child conceived with IVF. Two women were worried about being used as 'guinea pigs' and one other worried about the child's well-being if it was referred to as an 'IVF baby'. In retrospect, four women contemplated that 'desperation to get pregnant blinded me to the problems', and twelve said that they had no idea what they were getting themselves into as no one told them *really* what the procedure involved.

This comment leads to the almost unanimous response of the women in my study, that after waiting for an initial consultation for less than 1 month (thirteen couples), 3-6 months (13 couples), 12-18 months (8 couples) or longer, their first contact with the IVF programme had not been satisfactory (only five women said they had felt satisfied). Two women said:

> *Information was scarce. The first time was filled with excitement at the possibilities. Talks with the medical practitioner were brief purely because there was never an answer to our particular problem. "Everyone" was always guessing at possible solutions.*

And:

> *I was amazed at how easy it was to get on the programme. We were not offered any counselling, so I had to find help re emotional crisis myself. I felt like a Fresian cow ready to be experimented upon. I did not feel like a person after talking to Prof. X. The team aren't interested in people, only in science.*

With only eight exceptions, the first person the women met (invariably with their partners) was a medical doctor from the IVF team. One woman remembered:

> *He was nice but clearly seemed in a hurry. This was probably why he didn't explain much and instead made it seem as if everything was self-evident.*
>
> *He asked some medical information about our infertility — which I actually think my gynaecologist gave him — and then sent us away with three information sheets to make the next appointment for tests. It was only when we left the stifling and somewhat intimidating hospital atmosphere that we realised he hadn't asked a single question about ourselves — and also that we didn't know much more than before what IVF was all about.*

Four other women commented:

I felt the discussions were too quick and rushed through. I have always felt that further counselling was necessary but nothing altered. My suggestion of nurse-counsellor was "scoffed at".

I felt that the various options which were covered were explained fairly well — most of them I knew anyway, but I felt the amount of information given at once was too much to make decisions on immediately. I was very excited at the prospect of being a mother and this really clouded my ability to take information in.

I was horrified at the demands made on the woman and that I had no other women to talk to. I felt so isolated and freakish and lonely and an underdog or even a victim.

Now, I feel I did not ask enough questions about my own involvement. I certainly did not initially know enough of the workings of the female body and certainly was never prepared for the experience of IVF.

In some programmes the lack of acknowledgement of women's needs to acquaint themselves with the programme *and* their decision that, indeed, they were going to make this (next) step in their infertility 'career', has been recognised. However, what is now being offered as 'counselling' — or rather in many places by now is mandatory — is clearly a misnomer. One woman described it as follows:

When we finally [after 8 months] heard from the IVF clinic, we were asked to see an IVF counsellor first. With hardly any warming-up time he asked us if we had a good sex life and whether our marriage was happy. Of course we both nodded — obviously convincingly because he made a note somewhere on his form and then declared that we seemed emotionally stable and therefore were accepted on the programme! My husband and I both laughed about it afterwards. What a joke — who in their right mind after waiting so long would have even breathed a whisper of any difficulties?

Counselling, then, at this stage, and under these circumstances, has to be seen as tokenism. Conversely, there seems to be a real need for independent counselling which might help people with an infertility problem to put a halt to the 'insemination circus' as one woman called it, feeling both sarcastic and desperate but still agonising whether to try IVF for the third time. If such counselling were available and easily accessible, *some* women might decide *not* to embark on IVF. As one woman remembered:

> *In retrospect I realised it was a big mistake not to see a therapist before beginning IVF. I wasn't at all sure whether I had the energy to try again — and to cope again with disappointment. But I felt everyone was pushing me into it . . . gently but steadily . . . my husband, my mother, my best friend, even a girl at work whom I had told about it. I felt really caught . . . When we went to the initial counselling there was no space to say any of this. We were given the impression that it was a big privilege to be accepted — and we were — so we had to be grateful. I shut up and began three years of utter misery.*

Another woman commented:

> *The main feeling we had at the initial meeting was one of relief that it was at last happening. However, fairly quickly we felt that we were just part of the baby production line. The initial talks I feel are fairly useless as you are so happy and optimistic at that point it matters little what facts and figures are given to you. Actual details of the daily expectations while going through a cycle should have been given in greater detail.*

Given the severe dangers to the women from overstimulation of the ovaries — and possibly to their children from IVF (see Introduction), I was interested to know whether, at this initial meeting, there was a discussion of potential side-effects from the hormones during the IVF procedure.

Of the forty women, only nine said there was such a discussion. Moreover, if side-effects were mentioned at all, what was said ranged from 'Hormone levels will be affected' (1), 'Not a great deal of side effects' (1), 'Multiple births possible' (2), 'Lots of eggs will be produced' (1), 'dizziness/nausea' (2), 'weight increase' (1), and one woman was told 'Not to worry'.

As to mentioning the potential long-term side effects from the hormones, *only one woman out of the forty* answered in the affirmative. But what she had been told was:

> *It is a new science . . . we are not aware of potential long-term side effects.*

Ten women commented that they had been worried about possible effects from the drugs. Some of them looked for further information:

> *I was worried about the lack of information.I knew we were guinea pigs but I could not find any literature. Also, I desperately wanted IVF to work . . . and to believe the doctors who told me not to worry.*

Her words reflect accurately the difficult position women are in when they (and/or their partners) insist on having a child they cannot conceive naturally and turn to reproductive medicine for help. They trust the 'experts' will know best and act responsibly — and in the *women's* interest. The present research project, as well as other research (see Klein/Rowland, 1988), is cause for serious concern that, instead, women on IVF programmes are used as living 'test-sites' for fertility drugs and other seemingly limitless experimental research projects opened up by the thriving business of (in)fertility. *All* of this research depends in one way or another, on eggs or embryos that come from women.

I also wanted to know from the women in my study whether they had been asked what should happen with the extra eggs that might result from egg pick-ups, and what their decisions were. Twenty-two *were* asked and had to sign an official form of consent. Ten others said that some- questions were discussed but they could not remember signing anything. Five said no discussion, and three did not answer the question. The question whether extra eggs should be fertilised and the resulting embryos frozen was answered in the affirmative by thirty women and in the negative by three. Embryo freezing was not mentioned to four others and three others did not reply to the question. Twenty-seven women were asked whether they would donate 'spare' embryos for research, but only nine said yes (eighteen said no).

On the question of donating spare embryos to another infertile woman, out of the twenty-seven women who were asked only seven said yes (twenty said no). One woman specified her sentiments:

> *The thought of somebody else having our child . . . the thought of our baby running about, belonging to somebody else — it's too much to think about. I couldn't stand it. I'd rather destroy it than to donate to somebody else.*

The women's reluctance to donate 'extras' raises the intriguing question where the IVF scientists think they will be getting the substantial numbers of eggs and embryos that are required for embryo experimentation.[23]

In sum, the commencement period of IVF was on the one hand exhilarating and full of promises, but on the other hand highly frustrating. The lack of general information and counselling was experienced by most women. One woman summarises it as follows:

> *With hindsight I feel that the limited amount and content of the counselling that we received was fairly useless. It did little to prepare you for the actual physical and emotional demands placed upon you while going through the programme.*

Another woman said:

> *Being accepted on the programme raised wild hopes without any realistic information to back them up. Looking back I cannot understand why I did not see through it.*

The IVF Procedure

After a number of tests which vary greatly from clinic to clinic (ranging from rubella to vaginal swabs and smear tests, and from chlamydia to AIDS, including another sperm test from the partner), ovulation stimulation begins.

Clomiphene citrate — usually prescribed as Clomid — is the most frequently administered drug. Its Australian manufacturer, Merrill Dow, recommends 50 mg a day for five days to be commenced most frequently on the fifth day of the woman's menstruation (published in *MIMS*, 1987). Twelve women in my study were, indeed, on 50 mg Clomid a day, but twelve others were on 100 mg per day. Four women were given 150 mg daily. The administrations were usually for five days but two women remember six days on 100 mg and one woman said she was on 50 mg per day for a whole year. Merrill Dow recommends six courses of treatment as the longest time Clomid should be given. Another woman comments:

> *I started with one tablet a day but when the ultrasound revealed that my eggs did not grow properly I was told to increase the dosage up to four tablets [200 mg] a day. Then I was "cancelled".*

My ovary had swollen considerably and, despite reactions to release ripe follicles, no mature eggs were recovered.

The international medical research literature confirms the findings from this study: IVF practitioners do not always adhere to recommended guidelines for drug administration. An alarming fact given the increasing evidence that clomiphene citrate can present severe health dangers for both the women and, possibly, her future child (should she be among the very few for whom IVF works). There are also some theories that suggest that clomiphene citrate may stay in the woman's blood for at least six weeks after administration. If this is indeed true then, invariably, every woman who takes the drug for follicle growth stimulation will still have it in her system by the time the embryo is inserted and begins to develop in her womb.

Recent research also indicates that the drug may be the cause of chromosomal anomalies in a substantial number of stimulated eggs. The number of chromosomes, usually twenty-three in a human egg (or sperm) cell varies between five and twenty-five. If indeed these findings are the result of clomiphene citrate application, then this drug should be taken off the market immediately: it may not only be responsible for the approximately 80% of embryo transfers which do not work (see section Problems below), but also for the large number of miscarriages and the growing rate of birth abnormalities (in particular spina bifida); see Klein/Rowland, 1988, for a detailed discussion of fertility drugs used in conventional infertility treatment and IVF.

It is more difficult to assess how many — and what brand and dosage — of hormone injections were given to the women. Two women did not mention Clomid, but 'injections for ten days', probably hMG. As one woman said to me:

I never knew the name of the hormones they injected. We were not told. The number of injections and the day(s) of the cycle on which they were administered varied from patient to patient.

One woman reported sixty-eight hormone injections in five IVF attempts. Eight women mentioned Clomid and daily injections up to the time of the egg pick-up. Thirty-five women were given hormone injections before egg pick-up (hCG), twenty-eight of them 1 per day, seven 2 per day.

Many of the women — nineteen mentioned it specifically — felt adverse effects from the hormonal treatments. As one woman remembered:

> *I felt nauseous all day. Then I started having some strange blurred vision (no one had told me to expect this). Also I couldn't sleep and felt terribly depressed one moment — then next high up in the air.*

Another said:

> *When I think back, the thing that comes to mind immediately is sore breasts. I couldn't believe how much they hurt . . . I often wondered if I would ever be able to breast-feed.*

Nine women in my study reported developing cysts which necessitated the IVF treatment to be stopped. As one woman, who was on 100 mg Clomid for five days for 1 year, including ten days per cycle of hCG injections for 12 months, said:

> *I had to have yet another laparotomy when I was superovulated and developed very large ovarian cysts from clomiphene.*

Another woman — notably with a *low* Clomid dose (50 mg daily for three days, which indicates that there is *no* such thing as a *safe* dosage) said:

> *My body did not respond to hormone therapy in a positive way. I developed a cyst which caused more problems.*

And a third woman who had been given 50 mg Clomid for five days remembered:

> *My third attempt: sixteen eggs good size; when pick-up happened found cyst, lost eggs. No success. I was told my cyst had killed off my eggs but when I was unclear they told me they had drained my cyst and I could come in on my next cycle. After going home and having much pain I went back to my own doctor and was told I would have to go into hospital and have the large cyst removed. I could also lose one or both of my ovaries. I was very upset with this as it meant ten days in hospital, six weeks off work, and my*

fourth long operation. If I had taken my IVF doctor's advice who can say what would have happened?

The gruesome stories, unfortunately, continue with egg pick-up. One woman told me that following the laparoscopy she got a high fever and ended up in intensive care with a severe case of septicaemia: she could have died. Another woman, despite antibiotics provided as a preventative measure after egg-pick up via the vagina, developed a serious infection which inflamed her tubes and provided great cause for concern that *she might have been rendered infertile by the IVF procedure*: she was on the programme because of her husband's infertility. (Six months later, luckily her tubes seemed patent.)

Mixed with these stories of suffering actual bodily harm come tales of extreme tension, anxiety and stress. Asked whether she felt any side effects from the drugs administered, one woman said:

I felt so nervous and tense all the time I really wouldn't know. Somehow I managed to juggle work, housework, taking the kid [her child from a former marriage] to school and then rushing to hospital every morning for a whole month for blood tests, urine samples and ultrasound. And often my veins would not come up . . . I remember worrying so much that because of this it wouldn't work and I had to give up. You see it depends on each procedure; if part of the procedure doesn't work you are a failure again!

Another woman said:

It became a battle even doing part-time work. I could never let them know exactly when I was going into hospital and they naturally resented this. I felt that they would have preferred my resignation, but I didn't feel I could give up work even though my doctor had suggested this. But I thought, if I give up work and don't have a baby, then what will I have? What would I do with my time?

Many women felt during this time that they were just 'machines', just 'guinea pigs', 'on the assembly line', as one woman called the IVF programme. One woman said:

I was shocked at the number of women on the programme. I felt very unspecial, like a laboratory rat. I felt that my emotional needs were not being met by nurses and specially by my doctor. He hated me questioning his motives and would often pat my head and say "You don't need to worry about things like that." I felt I had to shut up or risk delay on the programme.

And yet another remembered:

I felt like a baby machine; no one was interested in me as a person. I was just a chook with growing eggs inside — and if they didn't grow properly then it was my own fault.

Others remembered — and were resentful about it — that they were treated with a lot of condescension by the IVF personnel. One of the fertile women remembered how she was chastised by a nurse for not producing more ripe egg cells:

Infertile women do better than you. What's the matter, can't you try a bit harder.

Many women commented that everybody always seemed in a hurry and had no time to answer questions. One woman summed it up:

No one ever talked to us about our experiences in the programme, I mean the psychological side of it. Doctors don't place a great deal of importance on you. For them you are just X, just another number.

Other women had very harsh words about the IVF doctors (see section Problems) but spoke highly of the nurses:

I really felt she [the nurse] understood how difficult it all was. Once I arrived in tears because I felt I just couldn't take it any longer. She sat me down with a cup of coffee and let me have a good cry — it felt wonderful. Finally, I thought, there is some one who understands me. It must be difficult working in the IVF ward.

And in some cases it was from other women on the programme that they got support, or — in as many as twelve cases — *gave* support to. As one woman put it:

I am basically a very happy person and was able to make the other girls feel better while we sat in the waiting room for what felt like hours with our full bladders. Once I was told by a sister that my good humour was very much appreciated. I felt good about that.

As many as half of the women in my study, that is twenty (out of forty) had to be 'cancelled' at least once during their IVF cycles. As already mentioned, sometimes it was because of ovarian overstimulation, but in eight cases it was because ovulation occurred naturally before egg-pick up began, so the eggs were lost and the women had to start all over again. Four women were angry because they had told the doctor or nurse they felt they were about to ovulate:

I said "Look, I know my body. I am feeling that I'm about to ovulate." They didn't believe me and I had the laparoscopy only hours later. When I woke up I didn't even need to ask. I knew there were no eggs — and there weren't.

Another of the fertile women commented:

I know my body really well. Always had very regular periods, always knew exactly when I would be ovulating. So I told them I wouldn't need a hormone injection to release eggs (I didn't want more hormones in my body!). They ignored me and insisted on the injection. I felt angry — and powerless.

And a third woman said:

I think IVF failed for me because of trying new drugs. My cycles were normal prior to IVF but once I started experimental treatments, they went their own way. IVF doctors and scientists fail to agree with me.

The majority of the women in my study — thirty-four — had egg pick-ups by laparoscopy, eleven had one oocyte collection via vagina and seven via bladder. The laparoscopies and transvaginal egg pick-ups were seen as manageable whereas four of the women undergoing the ultrasound-via-bladder technique (transvesical oocyte collection) said it was 'unpleasant'. The three others commented that it was 'very unpleasant'. One remembered:

During my third attempt Professor X said they would use a much better technique for egg recovery. I wouldn't need general anaes-

thesia and could watch what they were doing on the TV screen. So I was quite excited and looked forward to it. And then it hurt incredibly much . . . I winced and could not help twitching and moving my body. Prof. X was very annoyed and I heard him say to a nurse, "Knock her out, quickly" — which she did. I felt so bad afterwards but they found eight good eggs which consoled me a bit.

More than two-thirds of the women in my study (27) said they had some after-effects from egg pick-up. For fourteen it was feeling nauseous and dizzy from the anaesthetics, including a severe muscular tenseness, especially in the shoulder region. Seven others complained of abdominal discomfort, three got septicaemia. From egg pick-up via vagina four got an infection, and one said she got thrush. (Three others who did have a general anaesthesia with transvaginal pick-up also mentioned nausea and other reactions to the anaesthetic.)

Many women (18) commented on the excitement they felt when they were told the numbers of 'good eggs' that had been picked-up:

I couldn't believe it when they told me I was "superwoman": I had produced twelve really good eggs! I was so happy and proud of myself. Also I thought that out of twelve eggs some must fertilise and perhaps there would even be enough to have some frozen. I was over the moon with excitement.

Disappointment when there were no eggs was no less passionate:

I packed my belongings and felt really empty. All of a sudden this dreary hospital room was the place where I most wanted to be in the whole world. . . I was afraid to face the many empty hours in the week ahead. I had taken time off from work for the embryo transfer and a rest afterwards — what was I going to do with all the empty hours? What was I going to do with my life? Should I try again?

Another woman decided that 'enough is enough'.

Following the third ovum pick-up the gynaecologist told me my tubes were patent but my ovaries were bound by adhesions which prevented him from collecting the numbers of eggs which were there. He advised microsurgery via laparoscopy which would increase my chances of a pregnancy and allow more access to my ovaries, if a further ovum pick-up was to be done. However, I developed an ovarian abscess and septicaemia which necessitated three weeks in hospital — two further operations and removal of one ovary and tube, and four different types of intravenous antibiotics. When I recovered I realised my health and time with my husband was far more important than an endless endeavour to conceive a baby. At this stage, too, we were awaiting approval from Welfare Department to adopt a child.

For the women who continued, the wait began — waiting to hear whether the eggs had fertilised. One woman commented that she felt totally out of control just waiting:

It was my third attempt and they got ten eggs from me. They put four embryos back but I don't know what happened to the other six. They wouldn't really give us a proper explanation. They just said they were either immature or they weren't dividing properly or something like that. You really don't know what's happened to them.

Six other women complained that their eggs were 'lost' or 'mixed up' or were 'cooked', as one woman was told, which she took as overheating them during the time of fertilisation. Another woman remembered:

Well, one time when I was sitting there one of the girls went hysterical because one of the cleaners had pulled out the plugs on the incubator and her eggs were in there.

And another remembered that after she had been so positive because egg pick-up had resulted in eight eggs, she was shocked to learn that she should not continue:

When I was told after the third attempt that my eggs weren't good enough and that I should give up I was shocked and utterly devastated. I remained deeply depressed for more than a year and I was suicidal a lot of the time. I felt such an abysmal failure, a barren woman unable to give my husband a child and my parents their grandchildren. I had even failed technology.

For those whose hopes were once more up on the 'roller coaster of emotions' — as one woman called it — the embryo transfer was the next stage in the IVF procedure, and for most of them the final because for two-thirds it did not work (see also section Problems).

Eighteen women said the embryo transfer was 'manageable'. Eight felt it was 'unpleasant', mentioning pain (5), nervousness (4), discomfort (3e), and embarrassment (4). (Twenty-one women had been given Valium or another sedative before the embryo transfer.) One other commented:

> *The last two attempts I had epidural injections and it's very uncomfortable until you get the full feeling back in your legs.*

Four women said, 'It didn't bother me. The nurses were supportive and it was all fairly light-hearted.' One woman felt the procedure was extremely humiliating. She said:

> *I remember the first embryo transfer I had. At the time there were visiting doctors from IVF programmes around the world, and I happened to be one of the guinea pigs going in for the transfer on the day they were at the hospital. It is embarrassing enough lying there with your legs up in stirrups without a roomful of people staring at you and with a huge spotlight [theatre light] shining on your genitals! When my doctor said to me that after that day I would have an "international fanny" I was really annoyed at this remark, and the innuendo that I should somehow be thrilled at the prospect of being seen by all these international doctors.*

Another remembered her feelings as she was lying for four hours with her head tilted backwards:

> *I tried to relax, to feel positive, to have hope. But deep down I knew already it wouldn't work. I seriously considered getting up and leaving, but then you just don't. You keep doing what you are told.*

Four of the women resented the lack of concern by staff:

> *I wasn't impressed with the second try at all. The technician irritated me and I was virtually just left with my legs up and told I could go in half an hour!*

Asked how they experienced the time(s) waiting to know if they were pregnant, eleven women felt it was 'very unpleasant', ten said it was 'manageable' and eight ticked 'unpleasant' (no one ticked 'it didn't bother me').

One woman commented:

> *I could hardly stand it. I didn't feel I knew what to do — every move seemed dangerous, when driving, after every little bump I was convinced that was it, I've lost it.*

Another remembered:

> *I found it psychologically difficult trying to remain on an even level of not being either too optimistic or too pessimistic. It dominates all your thoughts and physical actions too.*

Problems

For eleven women IVF came to a halt because no eggs would ripen (three women had tried four times) or because they had to be 'cancelled' for fear of ovarian hyperstimulation. Egg pick-up was unsuccessful sixteen times including the instances mentioned by eight women who ovulated before pick-ups:

> *My first attempt ended in my ovulation being missed. This to me was devastating and made it very hard for my next time.*

Another woman said:

> *I was very annoyed at the doctors at the first attempt because they missed the egg pick-up. I knew beforehand but they wouldn't listen to me.*

In two instances the women's partners could not produce sperm, and in six instances there was something 'wrong' with the sperm. In another five instances something was 'wrong' with the egg. Eggs and sperm did not fertilise and develop in eighteen instances. Three women also mentioned that they were not given a clear answer as to what had gone wrong. In attempted pregnancies with frozen embryos, in four instances women were told that at least some of their embryos did not freeze properly; in another six cases the frozen embryos would not thaw undamaged. But for the majority of women — two-thirds of the women participating in my study — it was the embryos that did not implant themselves (in eighty-two attempts). Only six women got beyond this point, but for three of them, their pregnancies ended with an early miscarriage and for the other three with an ectopic.[24]

Asked to describe some of the feelings they had when IVF didn't work for them, one woman's statement stands for many similar ones:

> *I can't describe the feelings accurately, but I think it is akin to being grief stricken. Also the feeling of "Oh God, I've got to go through all this again in the next cycle." It is utter despair and extreme isolation. You feel you are a dismal failure.*

Other comments were:

> *It was a great disappointment for both me and my husband, seeing dreams dissolving and plans laughingly made, but half-believed, shattered. Even though you know that the success isn't high, you really hope that, and feel that, you will be among the lucky ones.*

> *I felt very giddy 10 minutes just prior to my periods. Cried all day — upset for myself as I had been thinking so positive, as everyone advised, that it was a shock to find I was not pregnant. Upset for my husband, for my mum who was hoping so much for her grand-child — looked after me when I came home from treatment and tried so hard. Bad headaches for a few days before any period. Emotional. Mourned my three "babies" that didn't survive and would never be. Felt it was such a waste — my little boy had been terribly upset by my absence for so long. My husband has been on his own for so long, all for nothing.*

> *I phoned in thinking I may be pregnant. I waited till the last minute. As so many phone in, the line is always busy, which makes it worse. I was told I definitely wasn't pregnant, that I would get my periods in the next few days. Initially I felt dumb knowing I wasn't pregnant, I think being told you are not really hits home. Then you have to pull yourself together to tell your husband and relatives.*

While having to hear, 'It did not work' was difficult to cope with at every stage of IVF, undoubtedly it was hardest when the woman got as far as the embryo transfer:

I cried and cried when I heard that the embryo transfer hadn't worked. Ever since they had allowed John and me to have a look at our embryos in the glass dish through the microscope I had really believed it. Yes, we could *have our own children, there they were. Mind you, I don't actually think of them as babies but these cells have the potential to become a baby, our own baby. For the first time that abstract hope "child" becomes real. And then all you get is this phone call. "Sorry, Mrs. H. See you next time." And you ache and ache but then sign on again because it seems you were so close, close as never before in your life. So you* had *to give it another try.*

It is the very fact of having produced a 4 or 8-cell live entity in the laboratory which for many people indicates that, 'this is real, this is *our* future child.' It may be an important reason why women who unsuccessfully tried many conventional infertility treatments said that when IVF failed it was much worse than anything else they had ever tried before. This is highlighted in the instances (six in my study) where the woman and her partner could, as a favour, go to the lab and have a look at their embryos under the microscope. This is a highly questionable procedure as it focuses on *technological* 'success' and ignores the fact that it is the *living* environment — a woman's body, specifically her womb — that in most cases seems to have different requirements for a successful pregnancy which ends with the birth of a *live child*, than such an artificially produced embryo seems to be able to fulfil. And because it gives people the feeling that they were 'almost there', it also ensures that many of the women immediately sign up for yet another try, that they feel they cannot quit.[25] As one woman put it:

I was very depressed and tearful but began to feel better when I was told I could come back on my next cycle. I was determined it would work next time: everything had gone so well. I also decided to quit my job to fully concentrate on IVF.

Another woman said:

I felt like a hamster on a wheel. I felt sick and tired and yet I couldn't get off it. I had become addicted.

This addiction, which in my view is largely constructed by the doctors (and often the nursing staff), as well as the women's social environment — 'try one more time' — contributes heavily to the woman's decision that she has no other choice than to go on. In my view this is not *choice*, as practitioners claim, when they say no woman is forced to continue, but amounts to *coercion* (see Klein, 1987a and Rowland, 1987b). As one woman said:

> *We were given five attempts and I tried them all although I had stopped believing it would work already after the second time. But at least I could then say "I have tried my very best."*

As the technological euphoria about 'artificially assisted' reproduction goes on, almost weekly a new variation of some old technology is praised as a 'promising breakthrough'! Unless the women manage to break out of the vicious circle, believing that perhaps with *one* more try and one more new technique they can get pregnant, it is extremely hard for them *not* to go on.

Having frozen embryos in storage may create another situation of coercion. The woman quoted next was not alone in mentioning that she believed she had to go back and 'use' her frozen embryos. Her case is special though because shortly after having been dismissed from the IVF program and being told that her husband and she had an insoluble infertility problem, she became pregnant naturally and gave birth to a child. She said:

> *You see, it's these frozen embryos. I've got frozen embryos from all three attempts. Now, I don't want them to be flushed down the sink, I don't want to give them for research and I don't want to give them to another woman. So what other option is there than go back? I know it sounds sick. Here I am feeling so angry about the programme, being totally sick of it, even having my own child, and yet, you know, you just plug on, on and on. Also, I must admit I feel quite maternal towards my embryos in the fridge — I used to tell my friends and they used to laugh — and I'm actually worried. I don't think we've had a bill for a while for storage fees. I'd be really pissed off if something had happened to them.*

All these forces keep women on IVF. Because they feel they must do it one more time they let themselves be exploited by doctors and biologists: as 'data' that walks 'voluntarily' into the lab, 'voluntarily' gives blood, and 'voluntarily' submits to yet another test, because perhaps it might be this one that will bring success. The desire for a child is thus exploited by those who need material to continue their research.[26] For many women though the feelings of desperation worsen with every new attempt.[27] Three women said:

On earlier attempts I was more optimistic, but as you have more failures your hope lessens. I handled the first three unsuccessful attempts quite well, but the last one I was rather depressed by it.

Each time the feelings became more acute because you knew that time was running out and maybe next time they would tell you not to bother coming back.

I got more upset after each attempt as I knew we had only limited finances so I would have to stop after five attempts. Time was running out.

In some cases, however, it is the doctors who advise the women to stop (this happened to nine women). One remembered:

I was emotionally drained and disappointed. No second attempt would be made without removing endometriosis which meant another major operation, after having had two already. Doctors advised against it.

Yet another could not understand why they were *not* allowed to continue.

My husband and I were summoned and told there was no point, we should give up. Prof. X couldn't give a convincing explanation as to why it was hopeless. We didn't seem to be so different from other couples we knew who also had idiopathic infertility. I was furious and couldn't help thinking that it was because I had asked [too] many questions. They prefer more submissive women.

Yet some other women *do* stop and I believe they deserve utmost respect for this difficult decision. One said:

Each time there was anticipated hope followed by devastation, crying, emotional upset, etc. After the third attempt I felt that I could not go through with all the emotional strain any more.

And another woman summed up her feelings as follows:

After attending hospital for two and a half hours one day, and being prodded and poked all that time, blood tests, ultrasound, needles, I eventually got off the table and said "Tell the doctor he can stick this up his jumper." I knew weeks of that would be untenable, especially after having to get up at 5.00 a.m. to travel two hours each way to hospital, and probably no baby at the end. What a joke. I feel so sorry for the women who have to use IVF.

Asked what made them finally decide not to try again, the women gave many reasons. Nineteen said 'I couldn't cope with the emotional stress any more.' One put 'I couldn't face the ups and downs' as her reason, and eight noted 'I couldn't bear the uncertainty.'

Physical risks were mentioned too: 'risks of infection' (6); 'wanted to withdraw from drugs' (5); 'surgery, *because* of IVF was too much' (3); 'miscarriage' (1); as well as problems with partner such as 'our future was up in the air' (14); 'stress on sex life' (8); 'his inability to cope with my misery while on the programme' (3); 'his inability to cope with negative results' (2).

Financial problems played a role too. 'It took all my wages' (4); 'it was a hard time for farmers; we couldn't afford it any more' (3). So did problems at work: 'ran out of sick leave' (6) and 'couldn't juggle work and IVF any more' (9). Thirteen women said they found a new interest (another job, art, business, sport, travel, study, living, etc). Fourteen became eligible for adoption, and three tried AID.[28]

For six women it was intensive counselling that they had begun during IVF (with a counsellor *not* associated with the IVF programme) that helped them in making the decision. Another said:

IVF meant only pain and disappointment. After all, I do have a daughter. I began reassessing my wishes.

Four women agreed that they did not believe in IVF any more. As one said 'I lost all trust in IVF.' Four other women said that even while they were still on the IVF programme, they had begun to accept infertility as part of their lives. As one put it:

Each day I woke up and said to myself "There is more to life than IVF. I must accept that we won't have our own child!"

The Time After IVF

Given the extremely stressful nature of IVF — because for many women it seems 'the last hope' — one would expect a well-developed counselling service already during IVF, but even more so *after*, since 90–95 out of 100 women will not be successful. Both assumptions are wrong.

Only four women reported some good counselling while on IVF, but even so, as one woman remembered:

I found it embarrassing. Also,we got a sheet saying the social worker was available for counselling. She was a really nice woman and I felt she had some understanding of why I felt so desperate. But she seemed always overworked so I felt guilty taking up her time. After all, I was only a childless woman. It wasn't as though I had cancer and really needed her support.

Another woman mentioned that she did not trust the counsellor associated with the programme.

She seemed OK, but I was wary of talking with her about my innermost doubts. How could I be sure she wasn't going to tell the doctors and then I'd be chucked off the programme?

In one Melbourne programme, perhaps due to criticism that there was no personal support for IVF 'patients', the women were requested to see their doctor each time a new phase in their treatment began. However, this visit needed to be paid for! One woman remembered angrily:

Like so much else on the programme I saw these "compulsory" visits as just another way [for the doctor] to make money. He charged $60 each time! Twice when I was there he didn't have a clue who I was because he had left my folder somewhere else. So all he said was, "How are you?" and, "Everything seems fine" — and not even that with feeling in his voice. He is a very strange man, rather up himself. He doesn't grow on one!

Some women were less courteous when it came to assessing the role of the IVF specialist:

He is a real pig — absolutely star-struck with himself, not interested in people only in science. He treated both my husband, who is a medical doctor, and me with such condescension. Incredible! And then I got the bill and it was horrendous. So I called him up and asked him about it but all he said was, "I am a superspecialist, that's what you have to pay for!"

One woman summed up the general feelings of many women when she said after IVF:

> *In hindsight I think there was no real contact with the doctors on the programme. No one you could ask questions and certainly there was no counselling or attention to the psychological aspects of participation in the programme, particularly coping with the failure afterwards. I am left with the impression that although the whole team are undoubtedly dedicated and conscientious, there is more concern with procedures and results and I couldn't help feeling like just another guinea pig.*

Another woman emphasised that once one is on the programme — and want to stay on it — one feels totally disempowered:

> *When I first came with my list of questions, Dr X patted me on my head and said, "Now don't you worry your little head off. We know what's best for you, so if you co-operate and stop worrying you'll have a good chance." Later, however, he stopped being so "nice" and once, when I complained about his assistant being too late for egg pick-up — which means that I had missed my chance that month — he commented sharply that, "Doctor's wives always cause trouble", and, "You want a child, don't you? If you do, then give up your job, stop being a problem and co-operate." So I felt I had to shut up or risk delay on the program.*

One other woman also commented that she couldn't stand the patronising tone she was subjected to by both nurses and doctors:

> *When some things didn't work doctors and nurses just lied. I think they did so in order to protect us from the harsh truth — which I couldn't stand. I felt I was being treated like a child at times or a very senile person who wouldn't understand anyway.*

The situation, however, gets worse when the IVF experience, in one way or another, has come to an end. Many women complained that there were no services available to cope with the feelings of desperation, let-down, ange, and — worst — not knowing what to do next. Only two women were offered counselling. Twelve others made an appointment with the doctor, but it could take a long time to happen. Said one woman:

> *No counselling was available but I did get a consultation with the IVF doctor. However, I had to wait two months for an appointment, which was annoying as the experience was no longer fresh in your mind. I found the lack of any kind of counselling an important matter which needed to be changed. A negative response on the other end of a phone from a virtual stranger, after you've been on tenterhooks for 2 weeks left me alone and down to deal with it the best way I could.*

Another woman commented:

> *We always had to see the IVF doctor about four weeks after treatment anyway. There is no support given or offered even at this visit. I found him very cold and clinical. If I treated my clients like that I wouldn't have any!*

Some women insisted on seeing their doctors immediately, with the result that they usually signed up for a further attempt straight away.

Almost half of the women (19) had felt ill since leaving the programme. Eight reported 'depression', 'emotionally unstable', three had an ovarian cyst removed, two complained of ovary pain and three of sore breasts. One woman had a hysterectomy, one abnormal cells in her cervix, one a lump in the neck, and one said 'I got shingles and nightmares.' Various others mentioned 'joint or muscle pains', 'eye problems', 'felt less fit and active', 'loss of hair', 'loss of libido' and 'failure to recommence ovulating'.

One woman remembered:

> *I felt very depressed for weeks following the failure of my second attempt. Emotional, unable to cope. Very lethargic, tired, headaches, bloated stomach, irritated. Continued to superovulate for at least two or three months afterwards. PMT effects tripled. The worst was the continual dizziness — began on the second day*

of the injections and only gradually improved. Even now, three months later, I still feel dizzy if I overdo things. For the first two months it was terrible. Three months after my first attempt I bled for three weeks and was very ill as I developed severe bronchitis at the same time. Now I have a rash — three months after my second attempt. The bleeding episode in June last year was very unusual for me — my GP said it was probably connected to the IVF treatment.

It is very clear from this study that no services are available for women who left IVF. Although there is a group in Melbourne called *IVF Friends*, their main aim is keeping 'failed patients' ' spirits up, always on the lookout for new technologies that, perhaps, might work. One of the women in my study commented:

I went only twice to their meetings. It wasn't what I wanted. I wanted to get away *from it, to find a new way of life. I was fed up with tales of miracles-to-be that never came true. Also, I couldn't stand their adoration of the doctors and scientists. I just don't think they are the wonderful people they make them out to be.*

Given the lack of services the women had to find their own ways of coping with life after IVF. It appears that almost half of the participants of this survey (eighteen women) began or continued counselling/therapy, some in connection with adoption, others while simultaneously trying to change jobs, return to study or find new interests.

Asked to think back on the time on the IVF programme and what image came to their mind immediately, these were the words that repeated themselves in thirty-four women's responses (five women did not respond to the question).

Emotional and physical stress, time consuming, emotions climbing and diving, great disappointment, hope and emotional upset, uncertainty, loneliness.

Other images were:

Unsympathetic doctors, who have no concern for you emotionally, playing with your body.

Extreme stress and a trial.

Blood tests, insensitive attitude of most medical staff.

A time of emotional and physical stress in chasing a very slim hope. I think it also affected other people around us so that on the last attempt we decided not to tell anyone.

Only *one* woman wrote down a positive image:

Excitement, happiness at a pregnancy. The kind and caring IVF sisters and sisters on the wards. The hugs and hand holdings to get me through the ectopic pregnancy. The women on the programme.

Asked to remember the *best* thing on the programme, sixteen women said 'other women', or, as one put it:

Finding out that I wasn't the only one, getting a lot of support from the other women on the programme.

One woman commented:

May I humbly write that maybe one reason for myself participating in the programme was that I was able to give support and loving to the other girls.

The other comments varied; nineteen women did not respond. Some of the answers were:

I can't think of one good thing.

I felt privileged to have taken part in a pioneering medical programme, and I learnt everything about my own body.

My husband and I learnt a great deal about each other.

Met other girls who understand what infertility is like, was given a chance — the closest I ever became to being pregnant and achieving my dream. Found that I was fertile — even with one ovary and all the problems I have I still did well on the programme, four eggs the first time and four embryos; five eggs the second time and three embryos.

That I learned that I was not the only one who could not have children. That there were worse cases than me. I learned to live with it.

I think I finally realised that we wouldn't have children naturally, so put my mind at rest.

The pregnancy.

I could say "I tried it" to myself, I've gone as far as I could.

Asked to remember the *worst* thing on the programme, *stress* was again one of the most frequently used words:

Extreme stress in waiting to be told and not knowing exactly when, and delay in knowing if the egg and sperm had fertilised into an embryo. It felt like an eternity. I was so anxious to know. Indifference and lack of sensitivity by nurses. Husband felt discounted quite often.

Other comments included:

Obviously the lack of baby at the end. The rest, whether unpleasant or not, was just accepted as a means to an end.

It was all pretty rotten.

It put a lot of strain on our marriage, family and friends. Our marriage nearly broke up a couple of times.

The doctor told me that I would never conceive. I went through a period of grieving which was completely unnecessary because we now have two beautiful daughters who were conceived naturally.

Having all these bloody vaginal examinations, all those probing questions, allowing myself to be subjected to two laparoscopies.

The ectopic.

The emptiness after being told it was unsuccessful. Blood samples being taken.

My cyst.

The feeling of failure, failure to yourself, your partner, family.

The feeling of utter failure at the end. The strain, emotionally, physically and financially. The blow to an already struggling self-image. The loss of my dream.

Not having a baby.

Every morning and late night blood tests and hanging around that waiting room.

Getting a pelvic abscess/infection from egg pick-up.

The second time when the whole procedure went haywire and I didn't even get down to theatre to pick-up eggs.

Thinking ahead to egg pick-up without anaesthetic — sounded inhumane and in fact the doctor was aiming to get 'numbers through', not treating people.

Trying new drugs and being given false hope by them.

Other people's expectations were so high. It was difficult enough coping with our own feelings but friends and some family thought it was just a matter of one trip to the hospital and I would be pregnant. Their ignorance was of no help, even though we explained over and over.

I also wanted to know how being on the IVF programme influenced the women's sense of identity.[29] Three women felt that it had no influence, and one said, 'It didn't really. I knew who I was and why I was there.'

Thirteen thought it had a negative effect similar to what one woman expressed when she said:

It tended to create a negative attitude in my own perception of myself. I thought of myself as a statistic.

Similar feelings came up in the next comments:

I felt that I was less than normal — after all my body didn't function properly. I felt very unimportant — just another childless woman. I felt I was reduced to being another pin cushion test case.

Six women put it down as a 'learning experience' as expressed in the next two statements:

I felt a bit like a number but I also learnt a lot about myself and how strong I can b. I began to think about how women are pushed around.

And one woman said that the IVF experience might have been helpful:

It may have accelerated my coming to terms with infertility — it may have just made it more painful — I find it hard to know.

As to their quality of life during IVF, the overwhelming majority — thirty-two women — said again 'full of stress'. Only five women put 'good', but without further comments. Three left the question unanswered.

In sum, then, women who underwent IVF and were unsuccessful have a painful story to tell of often long years of emotional distress, physical ill health — and no baby at the end.

DISCUSSION

Investigating women's experiences with IVF in this study concurs with women's experiences of IVF in other parts of the world (see Klein, ed. 1989). Women are experimental raw material for more and more variations of a basic technique which works only rarely. This study has also confirmed suspicions that women are *not* informed about potential adverse effects of the hormonal drugs given to them, and that the prescribed dosage as well as the hormonal cocktails — the mixtures of drugs administered — have in no way proved to be 'safe' but on the contrary can lead to serious health damage such as ovarian cysts (see Klein/Rowland, 1988).

The women's answers have also shown that in addition to the dangers from drugs, the IVF procedure itself is not without risk. Egg pick-up is not safe and can lead to infections which in turn may result in infertility in those cases increasing in numbers,[30] whereas it is *fertile* women who are on the programme because of their subfertile husbands. The same holds for cases of ectopic pregnancies, which is dangerous and emotionally draining event for all women, but particularly disturbing for fertile women who may lose a fallopian tube and be rendered (partly) infertile. We have also heard of fertile women's bodies thrown off balance because specialists didn't believe the women knew their own hormonal cycles and, we have heard of egg pick-ups being too late, because, again, IVF doctors did not listen to the women.

The story is a sad one and positive aspects are few: perhaps there was support from other women on the programme, sometimes helpful nurses, and in many cases a strengthened relationship with the women's partner after the marriage was almost on the rocks.

The women's verdict of the IVF doctors is almost unanimous. With very few exceptions they were described as 'cold', 'up themselves', 'only interested in science not people'; the comment about the absence of *meaningful* counselling before and during IVF is equally damning. And it is absolutely clear — and cause for great concern and worry — that the overwhelming number of women for whom IVF does not work are left without any counselling at the end. It thus seems reasonable to agree with what one woman said:

> *The only ones it works for are the doctors and scientists — not us!*

The most devastating finding of all is the close link between the stigmatisation of infertility and women's belief that 'they now *must* try IVF'; it might be 'the last hope'. Adult women without their own biological children are an anomaly in Australia (as in much of the rest of the Western world), and it takes a heavy toll to live within a family-centred society and *not* be able to have children naturally. It is thus not surprising — but no less disturbing — that once women have begun infertility treatment, the road to IVF in the 1980s seems almost unavoidable. Once the women are on IVF — with a few very courageous exceptions — it is understandable why they often continue to submit their bodies (and minds) to traumatic experiences, the consequences of which are far from being established.

Another striking feature of the women's answers are the *guilt feelings* that abound. Not only do women feel guilty for the infertility — even when it is their partner's — but when, once on the IVF programme, it doesn't work, they again believe that *they* have failed, rather than seeing it the way it is: that it is technology which has failed them bitterly. Its executors have a lot to answer for the ways they use women's bodies to experiment with techniques and methods that *fail* the great majority of their clients. IVF specialists also have a lot to answer for feeding women's negative feelings even more by telling them that their eggs are 'bad' and their wombs are 'a hostile environment' for their man-made embryos. All this reinforces feelings of worthlessness and low self-esteem in women who already are under great siege from a large part of society and pushed to the limit to produce children in order to be accepted as full human beings.

This study has doubtlessly confirmed that IVF is not in women's best interest: it doesn't produce babies and it often makes women seriously ill. What then can be done in order to spare women the many years of frustrating uncertainty, of stress and emotional pain — and still no baby at the end?

One clear outcome is that a society acting in the best interest of women's physiological and psychological well-being should do all it can to, firstly, prevent infertility, but, secondly, in those cases where it does exist, to ensure that involuntarily childless people are not stigmatised but are able to develop a strong — and accepted — self-identity as child-free people, including providing them with legitimate space (i.e. counselling services) to grieve over the wanted child. It is wrong to say 'women want IVF' and then offer them 'treatments' that make them ill and treat them like numbers and statistics — with a good dose of contempt for women and a failure to supply them with truthful information about the dangers involved in the procedures.

As long as 'childless' is seen by society at large as 'deficient' and 'abnormal', reproductive medicine and science will profit — in fact live off — the steady stream of women who have been made to believe that they must put themselves through the treadmill of baby-making, the roller coaster of exciting hopes and shattered illusions.

The tragedy lies in the fact that the women are determined to make a technology succeed which in the overwhelming majority of cases fails. What needs to be overcome is the continuing belief — in spite of their own experiences — that perhaps, one day, reproductive technology might work: for other women, or maybe even for themselves. While twenty-three women said they would never consider going back on the programme, one woman said she considered it 'rarely'.. Twelve women put 'I sometimes do', and four stated 'I often do'.

Again it is not the women who are to 'blame' for keeping up the hope, rather, the practitioners, groups such as *IVF Friends* and the media who, in spite of the evidence (i.e. continuing high failure rates), continue to spread the gospel of hope: 'Just try one more time, this new miracle drug or that revolutionary technique — and you will get your child'!

But perhaps the growing public awareness — in large part due to feminists' theoretical work and international campaigns — pointing to both the dangers inherent in reproductive technologies as well as the invasion of women's sense of self as autonomous persons with dignity and self-respect — will make it easier for women to reject IVF and to seek different ways of living happy lives.

People *truly* concerned with the well-being of women with a fertility problem can not continue to advise them using IVF. Especially after hearing the stories the Australian women told me in this survey and the ones I have collected from women from many other countries for my anthology (Klein, 1989b), encouraging a woman to try IVF seems like advising her to actively hurt herself — body and soul. To advocate the risks of trading an infection, an ovarian cyst, adhesions, burst ovaries, perhaps even cancer, and — should they be among those few who get pregnant — a spontaneous abortion, an ectopic pregnancy, a miscarriage, a stillbirth —

for no child at the end of years of laborious IVF treatments (not to mention the mental anguish), in my view is *not* compassionate understanding of the pain of infertility. Knowing what I do and not speaking out and actively trying to *stop* IVF as dangerous experimentation on women would make me an accomplice of the promoters of these procedures.

Rather, I believe that in addition to making room in society at large to accept women without children as 'normal', there have to be *active* attempts to give space to people with a fertility problem. Community and Women's Health Centres, for example, could offer self-help groups for women (and couples) to discuss their unfulfilled wish for a child of their own.[31] In this way women who have gone through IVF and have been unsuccessful could start support groups for one another. Hopefully, one outcome of such groups in addition to making it easier for the women to live with the knowledge that they will not have their own children, might be the offering of advice and counselling to other infertile women (and couples) *before* they have been drawn into the IVF treadmill. And eventually, I am sure, women who have undergone IVF will speak out: despite the social ostracism that this will invite from people who believe that medical authorities should not be criticised and/or that 'private' problems such as infertility should not be aired in public.

Gynaecologists should encourage women, who seek to investigate a fertility problem medically, to consider pursuing other options. For some this might still be adoption (although there are many problems associated with children who had to be relinquished by another woman, often under social or economic pressure), for others 'social' parenting, i.e. looking after the children of close friends or siblings. For yet others it might mean radically re-orienting their life goals and perhaps embarking on an exciting new educational or professional adventure. And close friendships with women provide one with another way of being nurturing and caring. In saying this I do not mean to make facile statements about 'getting over' one's infertility. As one woman who speaks for many said to me:

> *I can't really accept that I am infertile. Even now, two years after my last IVF attempt, I have moments when I deeply long for the child that never was. But because I have taken the time and space to rage, mourn and grieve over my unfulfilled desire I have accepted the fact that there are many things in life that one cannot have. So I have a good cry and get on with life — till the next time.*

I also hope that the voices of the large majority of the roughly 10% of infertile people in Western countries (precise figures are not known) who *did* expect and want a child but decided *not* to use IVF will become increasingly heard. As Rochelle A. Stackhouse wrote in the US Magazine Ms. (August 1988:12):

> *My husband and I have chosen, and are satisfied with our choice at the present, to "play the cards dealt us" — not to have children. In making that choice to live with our infertility as a family without children, we seem somehow abnormal to others we encounter, especially people with children. They constantly invade our privacy by asking why we don't adopt or try a new technology. Don't we like children? Are we prejudiced against children who don't share our genes? If society accepted us as we are, fewer of us would feel so pressured to have a child by any means, at any cost.*

The women in my study deserve a lot of respect for surviving the ordeal. My hope is that making public their experiences will help other women to say 'no' to reproductive technology. Above all, I hope their stories will contribute to exposing one more myth of beneficial medicine and science which, supposedly, is *for* people but, in reality, amounts to a cruel *modus operandi* based on trial and error in which it is women's lives that are strained to breaking point.

NOTES

1 It must be pointed out immediately that a large and increasing percentage of infertility problems are iatrogenic, that is, medically induced. Causes are pelvic inflammatory disease due to harmful intrauterine devices (IUDs, in particular the Dalkon shield which caused severe problems for millions of women worldwide). It also appears that there is a rather quick willingness on the part of medical practitioners to remove the fallopian tubes. In addition to iatrogenic causes of infertility, there is growing concern about health hazards, particularly at the workplace (i.e. workers being exposed to dangerous chemicals and metals, e.g. lead), as well as to pollution in general. And there is, in addition, the stress of living in the twentieth century where some other technological inventions,including the nuclear and chemical industry, that fundamentally change the climate (e.g. destroy the ozone layer), have brought us dangerously close to the edge of extinction. As a general rule (although there are no reliable statistics available) it is said that infertility worldwide is due one-third to female and one-third to male problems. The last third is said to be idiopathic, i.e. meaning the causes are not known. They include the above mentioned environmental factors plus, probably, specific physiological and psychological interactions between some women and men who try to have children. They also include women's reluctance to being mothers in a world in which mothering is still the least valued job. Being a mother usually means an extra full-time job for the woman in addition to her role as paid member of the workforce and as the unpaid emotional support for her husband and other family members.

2 While not usually calling their projects 'artificial womb', many research projects in animal reproduction concern themselves with the investigation of physiological and chemical processes that take part between the foetus/embryo and the mother's uterus. In some such projects it is stated that 'natural' conditions may indeed provide the growing embryo with more resources than needed (see Omar, 1984), thus inferring that an artificial womb could do just as well or even a better job than a natural uterus. A recent project that *does* mention the development of the artificial uterus in detail is presently being undertaken at the University of Louvain in Belgium. It is reported as 'Artificial Uterus: Culture of Oocytes and Embryos' (Henriet et al., 1985). Bovine immature oocytes and bovine and rat embryos are cultivated in an artificial uterus similar to a heart-lung-kidney system for up to 3-4 days. In addition, for humans it has been suggested by Peter Singer and Diane Wells that the artificial womb (ectogenesis) would be a perfect solution for feminists (and pro-life women) who could thus have abortions without guilt because their foetuses could still be carried to term in an artificial uterus and then offered

for adoption (1984:135). As a response to Singer and Wells, a whole article in the Australian journal *Bioethics*, No. 1 (James, 1987) was devoted to this subject. It is clearly an issue that is given a lot of attention and isn't a paranoic reaction on the part of feminists who fear that once the artificial womb was perfected, women would have lost the monopoly on birth. Indeed, in June 1988 the highly reputed US journal *Fertility and Sterility* reported the first case of ectogenesis. But it was a case with a twist. It wasn't the plastic incubator into which an embryo was placed in order to grow 'in man's image' — it was wombs taken from *three living women* — apparently cancer patients who had hysterectomies — into which spare embryos were placed, one of which then began its 'normal' development within a 52-hour lifespan. The uteri themselves were connected to so-called perfusion machines providing necessary nutrients and hormones mimicking early pregnancy. The experiment taking place at the Reproductive Medicine Unit at the Department of Obstetrics and Gynecology, the University of Bologna, Italy, 'was undertaken to obtain the first early pregnancy *in vitro* because future complete ectogenesis should not be ruled out' (Bulletti et al., 1987:991). Carlo Bulletti and his colleagues also reported that, 'The experimental design used in this project was previously approved by the Ethical Review Board' (p. 993).

The subject of maturing immature eggs *in vitro* is an even more burning one on the international research agenda. Borrowed clearly from similar research on cattle, before his death in March 1988 Britain's Patrick Steptoe — one of the 'fathers' of Louise Brown — was working on maturing immature eggs in a project entitled: 'Maturation of Immature Oocytes In Vitro' (*VLA Report*, 1987:19). By mid 1988 the 'egg fever' made news in Australia: 'Scientists set to "ripen" human eggs in millions' (Miller, 1988a). A scientist who has worked with programmes in the UK and been successful with egg maturation in sheep and pigs has now as his brief 'to perfect the procedure for human eggs' at the Centre for Early Human Development at Monash University. Calvin Miller reports that by using egg maturation techniques, Dr Jeremy Osborn 'predicts that the poor survival rates of fertilized eggs — less than 4 per cent for procedures' — an admission which is made rarely in the IVF context — 'will improve to match nature's 30 per cent survival rate.'

Dr Max Brinsmead, a reproductive physiologist at the University of Newcastle, Australia, also believes in the potential of maturing immature eggs to improve the success rates of IVF. Like Osborn, he is forthcoming with figures one usually does not hear from IVF specialists, such as 'about 95 per cent of 4-celled or 8-celled human embryos returned to the uterus fail to implant' — which is precisely what feminists have been saying for a long time (Miller, 1988b). According to Brinsmead, this low figure would be substantially increased if immature eggs could be collected and then matured *in vitro*. In his words (Miller, 1988b):

> Instead of stimulating the woman at the beginning of her cycle and collecting five or six eggs, we may be able to excise a small part of an ovary containing several hundred primordial follicles. We could then grow the follicles to maturity and harvest the eggs as they're needed.

This procedure, Brinsmead suggests, would result 'in a healthier patient and more receptive uterus at the time of the embryo transfer and could lead to a greater rate of successful pregnancies'.

While this is, of course, only a theoretical assumption, the idea of maturing immature eggs would, as Australian geneticist Dr Ditta Bartels rightly said (in Miller, 1988a):

> lead to a sudden surplus of literally millions of eggs . . . it will be like winning Tattslotto. All their dreams will come true . . . human embryos will become available for research.

Together with the method of freezing eggs the maturation of immature eggs would represent yet another giant step in the control and take-over of women's decision to have — or not to have — children, as well as their control over the circumstances and the time in their lives that they would like to have children.

Not only would human embryos be plentiful to allow for experimentation, but as has already been suggested with regard to the possibility of freezing eggs, a woman might be coerced to have her eggs frozen at an early age when they are still 'good'. In other words, before the adverse effects of a polluted environment including hazardous work conditions or cancerous chemicals have deteriorated the 'quality' of her eggs.

It is not the prevention of health hazards at the workplace that is targeted; it is the prevention of 'living a normal life' that is sought, a life-hating philosophy which places little importance on the well-being of its *living* population — women and men — and is instead only concerned with the controlled survival of the human species — of molecule-machines — whateve the price.

Seen in this light, Dr Brinsmead's statement that the successful technique of maturing immature eggs may be applied to extracting egg follicles from a *foetus* may not be that surprising: 'A foetus which is not even born could ultimately have children', he says and explains (in Miller, 1988b):

> By the 14th week a foetus contains its full complement of 100 million oocytes surviving in the neonate [newborn]. Thus, terminated foetuses or non-surviving neonates could theoretically become egg donors.

Once this technique is perfected, *any* ovary of *any* woman will do — young or old, fertile or infertile. It will be possible to mature the egg cells in the laboratory, fertilise them with sperm (easily available) and implant them in, perhaps, hired breeder women (e.g. poor women from developing countries who are desperate for the little money and decent food for the nine month period of their pregnancy).

3 Reporting what they call 'crude live births', the British figures established by the Voluntary Licensing Authority (VLA) were 8.6 per cent for both 1985 and 1986 (*VLA Report*, 1988, p. 19). Australian estimates per IVF treatment cycle for 1986–87 were similar: 8.8 per cent of live births (Batman, 1988b, p. 3; these include also on-going pregnancies over 20 weeks). Not reflected in these numbers are the significantly increased number of children born prematurely (26.9 per cent for 1986, National Perinatal Statistics Unit, Australia 1987) — who are most frequently delivered by caesarian section (43.9 per cent instead of 15–18 per cent for 'natural' pregnancies in Australia in 1986 (Stanley, 1988) and therefore of low birth-weight and in need of extra neonatal care. Nor do they highlight the high proportion of multiple births — just under one-quarter of all IVF/GIFT pregnancies in Australia (NPSU, Tables 30 and 39) and 24 per cent reported for England in 1988 (*VLA Report*, 1988, p. 21). The high proportion of children born with abnormalities is also cause for serious concern. These are mostly neural tube (spina bifida) and cardiac problems (transposition of the great vessels): 2.2 per cent compared with 1.5 per cent from 'natural' pregnancies for Australia. Taking these cases into account (and the premature children needing intensive neonatal care), the Australian government report concludes that the success rate for an 'unproblematic live birth' is 4.8 per cent (Batman, 1988b, p. 3).

4 Among them in English see the books by Arditti et al, 1984; Corea, 1985a; Corea et al., 1985; Spallone and Steinberg, 1987; Scutt, 1988; Klein, 1989a; in German *Beitraege* 14, 1985; Bonner Kongressdocumentation 1986; Fetz et al., 1986; Zipfel, 1987; Weikert et al., 1987; Roth, 1987; Pauritsch et al., 1988 as well as numerous journal articles, e.g. Crowe, 1985; see Further Reading for details.

5 For an excellent discussion of foetalist *vs*. feminist see Janice Raymond, 1987.

6 See Linda Bullard, 1987, who also mentions the application of biotechnology in genetic warfare. See also Klein, 1989b, for an overview of genetic engineering.

7 The frightening similarities of many of the 'new' reproductive technologies (including the expanding range of prenatal tests such as pre-implantation diagnosis) to the old eugenicist dictum of *heilen und helfen* (heal and help) which in reality means *auslesen und ausmerzen* (select and eradicate)

are most succinctly articulated by German feminists. See in particular Heidrun Kaupen-Haas (1988), who links today's research in reproductive technology with research projects into human (female) reproduction conducted in Nazi Germany.

8 For a discussion of reproductive technologies and contraceptives/sterilisation/abortion as two sides of the same coin, see Balasubrahmanyan, 1984; Klein, 1985; Hartmann, 1987; Klein, 1989b. It is very important to see clearly the connections between supposedly 'helping' some women to have a child while 'helping' others not to conceive as the other side of the coin: both forms of (harmful) control executed by a third party — the state and/or the medico-scientific profession, backed up by a capitalist profit-seeking industry over women's reproductive capacities.

9 See Gena Corea, 1985b, for a description of the DES story; Direcks and Holmes, 1987; Direcks, 1987, for some of the possible links between DES and cloiphene, and Klein/Rowland, 1988, for an overview of clomiphene citrate and other hormonal cocktails.

10 Doing research on a group that is currently undergoing the procedure which the research project is investigating, always contains two specific problems as to the conscious and unconscious readiness of the participants to speak openly about their experiences: a) to be wary about saying anything that might jeopardise their participation in the project/procedure they are involved in, and b) an almost imperative necessity to maintain a positive attitude to what they are doing for their own sake. Specifically, for IVF, this means that women who *are* involved in IVF have said to me that they would rather not talk about the problems involved *which they could see*, but 'go ahead with it, give it a go and hope for the best' (personal communication, 1987). In the tradition of doing feminist research (Klein, 1983 and 1986) it seems crucial that we respect these dilemmas as much as possible, because otherwise we might be in a similar position as the increasing number of non-feminist researchers who, on the look out for 'data', exploit these already highly vulnerable groups; see for example the German psychoanalyst Peter Petersen (1985) who, whilst being against IVF, puts the full blame for its existence on the women who — supposedly want it because they are 'pathological' and display 'emotional passivity' and 'a dearth of feelings' (p.8). Christian Bachman, a Swiss author, goes even further and predicts that children conceived by IVF will have a hard time because of their emotionally insecure mothers who needed a child for their 'narcissistic equilibrium' (1987:22). In addition to using women as 'data', such (male) interpretations do not acknowledge the societal pressures on women to become mothers (including the often strong push from their male partners to have their 'genetically own' child). They conveniently blame women for 'wanting it' and thus create a

paradoxical mixture of contempt and pity for women on IVF programmes, indicating that they are 'neurotic', thus bestowing upon themselves the right to use 'these women' as experimental fodder. My survey indicates — as I will elaborate in the main text — that women who undergo IVF are 'ordinary' women whose determination in life to have a (or another) child does not make them more or less 'neurotic' than other people who would try everything to have a specific desire fulfilled.

11 I am grateful to a Humanities Grant from Deakin University for financial assistance to run these advertisements.

12 I continued this research project upon my return to Australia in September 1987 as Post-Doctoral Research Fellow at Deakin University, Geelong.

13 *Infertility: Women Speak Out About Their Experiences of Reproductive Medicine* (Pandora Press and Allen & Unwin, 1989).

14 I am also grateful to the affiliates of FINRRAGE, the Feminist International Network of Resistance to Reproductive and Genetic Engineering, among them in particular Lene Koch, Denmark; Alison Solomon, Israel; and Ute Winkler, West Germany.

15 I also thank Mary Rice for her assistance with the questionnaire analysis, Arlette Eastgate for typing many of the answers to the open-ended questions, as well as Judy Barber, Nancy Stefanovic, Jane Veale, Bev Bartlett and Jan Wapling for secretarial support at Deakin University during my time as Georgina Sweet Fellow.

16 I think that this is one of the reasons why even those women who were very critical of IVF when they told me their stories do not want to speak out against it in public. Much as I would like them to make public the horrendous stories they have told me — and I have asked some women repeatedly to do so — their decision to remain silent must be respected. The pro-IVF lobby — doctors and their spokeswomen — would most likely try to malign them by portraying them as 'embittered, frustrated' women. The press would love the dispute, and the women's personal lives — including their families' — would be exposed. It appears that they are not willing to become 'public property'; partly because of the stigma attached to admitting that one is infertile, partly because they don't want another upheaval in their lives. I do hope, however, that this silence will soon be broken and that a group of women, together, will have the courage to come out and tell the *real* story of IVF!

17 In my analysis I am using the concept of 'heteroreality' developed by US philosopher Janice Raymond (1986) positing that we all live in a

system — patriarchy — in which men's needs and interests try to determine women's realities albeit in many different ways depending on culture, class, etc. It is my contention that IVF, and reproductive and genetic engineering in general, are prime examples of this desire to control, conquer and rule over living material — women's bodies (and souls) included.

18 A group of concerned French academics, including scientists, are preparing a statement to be published in early 1989 in which they condemn IVF as a *violation of human rights* according to the UN Charter of Human Rights (Corea, personal communication, 1988). IVF doctors in France are now predominantly using Buserelin and other LH-RH (luteinizing hormone-releasing hormone) analogues in order to 'harvest' mature eggs. This drug puts women into a chemical menopause by desensitising the pituitary (an important hormone centre in the brain). Once the women's hormonal cycle has stopped, they are given very high doses of hMG (human menopausal gonadotropin; a frequently used brand is Pergonal) which re-stimulates follicle growth. Unfortunately, before the cycle stops there can be a huge LH-RH surge leading to dangerously hyperstimulated ovaries which, according to some French doctors, are the worst they have ever seen (Laborie, 1988). Buserelin is a highly experimental drug; in Australia it is not (yet?) officially used on IVF programmes. It is, however, used in trials (see Batman, 1988a) and as a drug for fibroids and prostate cancer.

19 It is of course true that in other western societies too, women are in general expected to have children. Pro-natalist State interventions such as payment of a *Muttergeld* (motherhood allowance) in West Germany — a pitifully small amount of money — is aimed at halting the continuously falling birthrates. Nevertheless, I have come to believe that in Australia the sense of 'family' — which is invariably defined as husband, wife and at least two children — is still more pervasive than in European countries or the USA. This may be an important reason why Australian IVF research has been able to proliferate, helped by the media — especially the women's magazines — which praised (and continue to do so) IVF as a miraculous cure-all which every woman with an infertility problem now *must* do. A notable exception was a critical story on IVF by Leta Keens in the *Australian Women's Weekly* (June 1988).

20 These problems would appear to be different for the ten women who already have children from a previous marriage or prior to the fertility problem in the present relationship. However, in my study they appear to be more similar than expected: the desire to have another child with a different person — and the emotions of feeling 'lost' by not being able to do it — does not seem to be mitigated by an already existing child. Some women also indicated clearly that they were afraid their second husband

(usually a younger man) would leave them for a younger woman if they did not 'give him his own child'.

21 More and more perfectly functioning fertile women (I do not wish to use the term 'normal' which I consider an insult to women with an infertility problem since it declares them 'abnormal') undergo the IVF procedure: there is a rapid increase in subfertile men whose partners are then directed to the IVF programmes where they serve as experimental subjects for new techniques (i.e. the microinjection technique). From France the figures are 16% for 1986–87 (Laborie 1988), but an Australian doctor recently said that as many as 30% of his clinic's 'patients' came because of male infertility (Ferber, personal communication, 1988). Given the health dangers as well as the emotional stress involved in IVF I think it is ethically highly questionable to use these women as 'living laboratories' (Rowland, 1984) for a totally experimental method when 'conventional' IVF issued (where the subfertile man's sperm is placed with the egg cell in a petri dish) the high percentage of fertile women certainly boosts the low success rates — much wished for by IVF specialists!

22 The media have a lot to answer for in promoting the *false* view the general public has about IVF. Internationally, journalists have advertised doctor-centred, glamorous images of 'happy mothers' and worthy IVF 'fathers' — all men in white lab coats — who can now surpass nature and play God. No word about problems, no word about the fact that IVF only works for a tiny minority (5–10%), and certainly no word about the trauma the women go through while on IVF — and after. Joachim Marcus-Steiff (France) has written an excellent article on this topic which holds true internationally. Using a good wordplay he discusses how 'medically' assisted procreation has also been 'mediatiquement (by the media) assistée' (Marcus-Steiff, 1987). It appears that in the last 2–3 years, there *has been* some more critical reporting on IVF (e.g. in *The Age*, Melbourne), but it in no way balances the soppy nature and hope-raising stories in other publications.

23 The amendment to the *Infertility (Medical Procedures) Act (Vic.) 1984*, which was proclaimed in July 1988, specifies that embryo research up to 22 hours may only be conducted on embryos from couples on programmes. If indeed women on IVF programmes who are reluctant to donate eggs or embryos *are* to be the only legitimate egg/embryo donors, then it seems that additional (moral) pressure will be put on women to donate spare eggs/embryos. But then, of course, there is a lot of on-going research on maturing immature eggs *in vitro* (see Note 2), so the problem of the scarcity of eggs could soon be solved by technological 'progress'.

24 Dr Fiona Stanley of the NHMRC Research Unit in Epidemiology and Preventive Medicine, at the University of Western Australia, writes in the

Medical Journal of Australia (May 2, 1988) that in 1986 of the IVF pregnancies that began — which is only about 20% of successful embryo transfers, perhaps even less — 42.5% ended in preclinical abortion, ectopic pregnancies, spontaneous abortion and still birth (p. 425).

25 Kirsten Kozolanka, a Canadian woman with a fertility problem, reflects movingly on the painful dilemmas that result from feeling trapped on the medical treadmill once one has begun the process of investigating a fertility problem. She calls it 'the choice that isn't': you don't want to be a 'quitter' (in Klein, 1989a). This is why groups such as the *IVF Friends* are no help once the women have reached the point where they wish to stop IVF. On the contrary, their fierce determination not to give in, to keep on trying and trying, prevents them from helping women to make the break and leave the IVF programme.

26 French biologist Jacques Testart, who was the 'lab father' of the first French IVF child in 1982 but who has since publicly distanced himself from human IVF research, deplores the fact that working with monkeys — which he does now — is much harder than with women. Monkeys, he said, needed to be fed, kept good humoured and it was very hard getting any co-operation for the research. Women, on the other hand, would do all this voluntarily. I am sure his sentiments are shared by many IVF practitioners. They reflect a deep-seated contempt of women who, it seems, because they want a child, can be used for any experiment that needs to be done (see Klein 1987b).

27 For some it remained the same. One woman said: 'It was the same feeling of despair, that you would never be successful, that it was all be-cause of your fertility problem; it made you very determined to keep going.'

28 It is truly amazing that three women underwent IVF first before trying AIH or AID given the much less intrusive nature of artificial insemination and its much higher success rate!

29 Seventeen women did not respond to this question, the lowest number of respondents to a question. Of course one could say that the question about self-identity was on page 32 of the questionnaire and that they were sick and tired of it at that stage. However, I tend to speculate that it has to do with the general recognised *lack* of women's sense of self and hence identity as has been clearly established by many writers (see, among others, Rowland, 1988). I do not mean to set up women who go through IVF as a 'special' group — women in general appear to be rather low on self-esteem. But I think the long and traumatic IVF experience in which women again believe it is *they* who fail (rather than *technology* failing them) can add to the dwindling sense of self and may be one reason for the

many blanks in response to the question about their sense of identity.

30 In 1987 Alan Trounson said, 'I believe that eventually more than 50% of our patients entering IVF will have "male factor" as the primary reason for their infertility (Trounson, 1987; in Bartels, 1988:17). Using the bodies of *fertile* women might boost the success rates, clearly a desirable outcome for a technology with increasing failure rates for infertile women. But it appears ethically highly questionable to submit fertile women to the physically dangerous and emotionally draining IVF procedure when it is their partners who have the fertility problem.

31 Such groups are already offered — and highly successfully — in a number of Women's Health Centres in West Germany; e.g. Frankfurt and Berlin. See Winkler and Schönenberg in Klein, 1989b, for a detailed description of the different options (self-help groups; counselling, etc.).

Also, FINRRAGE (Feminist International Network of Resistance to Reprtive and Genetic Engineering), in existence since 1984, monitors develo reproductive technology and their impact on women's lives. The Austn chapter (Melbourne) also produces a quarterly newsletter and would be happy to put women who want to discuss fertility problems (or leave IVF programmes!) in touch with one another.

The address is FINGRRAGE, P. O. Box 248, East Kew, Victoria 3102.

REFERENCES & FURTHER READING

Arditti, Rita; Klein, Renate Duelli and Minden, Shelley (eds). 1984. *Test-Tube Women. What Future for Motherhood?* Pandora Press, Boston and London.

Bachmann, Christian. 1987. 'Vom Sinn der Unfruchtbarkeit und vom Stress der uebermaechtig ersehnten Kinder.' In: *Tages-Anzeiger Magazin Zuerich*, Nr. 9, 28 February 28:16–23.

Balasubrahmanyan, Vimal. 1984. 'Women as targets in India's family planning policy.' In: *Test-Tube Women*, Arditti *et al*: 153–164.

Bartels, Ditta. 1987. 'High failure-rates in *in-vitro* fertilization treatments.' *Medical Journal of Australia* 147:474-475.

——. 1988. *In Vitro Fertilisation in Australia.* Submission in Response to Commonwealth Perspectives on IVF Funding.

Batman, Gail. 1988a. *In vitro Fertilisation in Australia.* Commonwealth Department of Community Services and Health, Canberra, Australia.

——. 1988b. *Commonwealth Perspectives on IVF Funding. A Discussion Paper.* Commonwealth Department of Community Services and Health, Canberra, Australia.

Bowles, Gloria and Klein, Renate Duelli (eds). 1983. *Theories of Women's Studies*. Routledge and Kegan Paul. London and Boston.

Bullard, Linda. 1987. 'Killing Us Softly: Toward a Feminist Analysis of Genetic Engineering.' In: *Made to Order*, Spallone and Steinberg (eds): 110–119.

Bulletti, Carlo *et al.* 1988. 'Early human pregnancy *in vitro* utilizing an artifically perfused uterus.' *Fertility and Sterility* 49 (6):991–996.

Cabau, Anne. 1986. 'Les Dangers des Inducteurs de l'Ovulation.' In *La Lettre du Gynecologue* 45, May 1986:2–4.

Carter, Marian E. and Joyce, David N. 1987. 'Ovarian Carcinoma in a Patient Hyperstimulated by Gonadotropin Therapy for In Vitro Fertilization: A Case Report'. In: *Journal of In Vitro Fertilization and Embryo Transfer*, 4(2): 126–128.

Corea, Gena. 1985a. *The Mother Machine*. Harper and Row, New York.

——. 1985b. *The Hidden Malpractice*. Harper and Row, New York.

—— *et al.* 1985. *Man-Made Women, How New Reproductive Technologies Affect Women.* Hutchinson, London/Indiana University Press, Bloomington (1987).

—— and Susan Ince. 1987. 'Report of a Survey of clinics in the USA'. In: *Made to Order*, Spallone and Steinberg (eds): 133–145.

Conseil du statut de la femme. 1988. *Sortir la Maternité du laboratoire.* Gouvernement du Quebec, Canada.

Crowe, Christine. 1985. '"Women Want It': *In Vitro* Fertilization and Women's Motivations for Participation' In: *Women's Studies International Forum*, 8(6): 547–552.

Du Bois, Barbara. 1983. 'Passionate scholarship: notes on values, knowing and method in feminist social science'. In: *Theories of Women's Studies*. Bowles and Duelli Klein (eds): 105–116.

Die Gruenen im Bundestag, AK Frauenpolitik & Sozialwissenschaftliche Forschung und Praxis fuer Frauen e.V. Koeln. (Hrsg.) 1986. *Frauen gegen Gentechnik und Reproduktionstechnik*. Verlag Koelner Volksblatt.

Direcks, Anita and Holmes, Helen Bequaert. 1986. 'Miracle Drug, Miracle Baby.' In: *New Scientist*, November 1986: 53–55.

——. 1987. 'Has the Lesson Been Learned? The DES Story and IVF'. In: *Made to Order*, Spallone and Steinberg (eds): 161–165.

Ehrenreich, Barbara and English, Deirdre. 1978. *For Her Own Good: 150 Years of the Experts' Advice to Women*. Anchor Press/Doubleday, New York.

Fetz Anita. Koechlin Florianne und Mascarin Ruth (Hrsg.) 1986. *Gene, Frauen und Millionen*. Rotpunktverlag, Basel.

Gomez Dos Reis, Ana Regina. 1987. 'IVF in Brazil. The Story Told by the Newspapers.' In: *Made to Order*, Spallone and Steinberg (eds): 120–132.

Hansen, Friedrich und Kollek, Regine. 1985. *Gen-Technoloqie. Die soziale Waffe*. Konkret Literatur Verlag, Hamburg, 1985.

Hartmann, Betsy. 1987. *Reproductive Rights and Wrongs: The Global Politics of Population Control and Contraceptive Choice*. Harper and Row, New York.

Henriet, L *et al.* 1985. 'Artificial uterus: culture of oocytes and embryos'. Abstract 89 in section *In vitro* fertilization and embronic growth. 1st Meeting of the European Society of Human Reproduction and Embryology, June 1985: Bonn. 32.

Holmes, Helen Bequaert, Hoskins, Betty and Gross, Michael (eds). 1981. *The Custom-Made Child? — Women-Centered Perspectives*. Humana Press, New Jersey, USA.

Homans, Hilary (ed.). 1985. *The Sexual Politics of Reproduction*. Gower Publishing, Aldershot, UK.

James, David K. 1987. 'Ectogenesis: A Reply to Singer and Wells'. In: *Bioethics* 1(1):80–99.

Kane, Elizabeth. 1988. *Birth Mother. The Story of America's First Legal Surrogate Mother*. Harcourt Brace Jovanovich, San Diego.

Keens, Leta. 1988. '10 years on IVF: Is it worth it?' *Australian Women's Weekly*, June 1988.

Klein, Renate Duelli. 1980. Between Progress and Backlash: Exploring the Attitudes of Undergraduate Women at UC Berkeley Towards Feminism, The Women's Movement and Women's Studies. Unpublished BA thesis (Highest Hons) Women's Studies Program, UC Berkeley, California.

——. 1985. 'What's 'New' About the 'New' Reproductive Technologies?' In: *Man-Made Women: How New Reproductive Technologies Affect Women*, Hutchinson London/Indiana University Press, Bloomington. (1987):64–73.

——. 1986. *The Dynamics of Women's Studies: Its International Ideas and Practices in Higher Education*. Ph.D. Dissertation. University of London, Institute of Education, UK.

——. 1987a. 'Where Choice Amounts to Coercion: The Experiences of Women on IVF programmes'. Paper presented at 3rd Interdisciplinary Congress on Women, Dublin, Ireland, 6–10 July 1987.

——. 1987b. 'When Medicalisation Equals Experimentation and Creates Illness: The Impact of the New Reproductive Technologies on Women. In: *Sortir la Maternité du Laboratoire*, Government of Quebec, Canada.

——. 1988a. Segen oder Fluch? Reproduktions– und Gentechnologie aus feministischer Sicht. In: *Kinder machen. Strategien der Kontrolle weiblicher Fruchtbarkeit*, Gertrude Pauritsch *et al.* (eds) Wiener Frauenverlag, Austria.

——. 1988b. 'Biotechnology and the Future of Humanity'. *Women's Worlds. ISIS-Wicce.* March (Part I) and June (Part II).

——. 1988c. 'Genetic and Reproductive Engineering: The Global View.' In: *The Baby Machine. Commercialisation of Motherhood*, Jocelynne Scutt (eds), McCulloch, Melbourne:235–273.

——. (ed.). 1989a. *Infertility. Women speak out about their experiences of reproductive medicine.* Pandora Press, London; Allen & Unwin, Sydney.

——. 1989b. 'Resistance: From the Exploitation of Infertility to an Exploration of In-Fertility.' In: *Infertility. Women Speak Out*, Klein (ed.): 229–295.

—— and Robyn Rowland. 1988. 'Women as Test-Sites for Fertility Drugs: Clomiphene Citrate and Hormonal Cocktails.' *Reproductive and Genetic Engineering: Journal of International Feminist Analysis* 1(3): 251–273.

Kollek, Regine; Tappeser, Beatrix und Altner, Guenter (Hrsg.) 1986. *Die ungeklaerten Gefahrenpotentiale der Gentechonologie*. J. Schweitzer Verlag, München.

Laborie Francoise. 1988. 'News from France and Elsewhere'. In: *Reproductive and Genetic Engineering: Journal of International Feminist Analysis 1* (1): 77–85.

Lasker, Judith N. and Borg, Susan. 1987. *In Search of Parenthood and Coping With High-Tech Conception*. Beacon Press, Boston/Pandora Press, London 1989.

McNeil, Maureen *et al.* 1989. *The Social Dimension of Reproductive Technologies*. Macmillan, London.

Marcus-Steiff, Joachim. 1987. 'La procreation mediatiquement assistée.' In: *L'Ethique autrement* No. 93, October 1987.

Mies, Maria. 1983. 'Towards a methodology for feminist research.' In: *Theories of Women's Studies*, Bowles and Duelli Klein (eds):117–139.

Miller, Calvin. 1988a. 'Scientists set to "ripen" human eggs in millions.' *Herald*, Melbourne, June 29.

——. 1988b. 'When a foetus is a mother.' *Australian Doctor*. May 27.

Oakley, Ann. 1981. 'Interviewing Women. A Contradiction in Terms.' In: *Doing Feminist Research*, Helen Roberts (ed.). Routledge & Kegan Paul, London.

Overall, Christine. 1987. *Ethics and Human Reproduction. A Feminist Analysis*. Allen & Unwin, Toronto and Sydney.

Petersen, Peter. 1985. 'Expression of Dissent Concerning the Final Report of the Working Group on IVF, Genome Analysis and Genetic Therapy.' In: *Benda Report*. Bonn, West Germany.

Raymond, Janice. 1986. *A Passion for Friends. Towards a Philosophy of Female Friendship*. Beacon Press, Boston; The Women's Press, London.

——. 1987. 'Fetalists and Feminists: They Are Not The Same'. In: *Made to Order*, Spallone and Steinberg (eds):58–66.

Reinharz, Shulamit. 1983. 'Experiential analysis: a contribution to feminist research'. In: *Theories of Women's Studies*, Bowles and Duelli Klein (eds):162–191.

Roth, Claudia, (Hg). 1987. *Genzeit Die Industrialisierung von Pflanze, Tier und Mensch, Ermittlungen in der Schweiz*. Limmat Verlag, Zuerich.

Rowland, Robyn. 1984. 'Reproductive Technologies: The Final Solution to the Woman Question?' In: *Test-Tube Women: What Future for Motherhood?* Arditti et al. (eds): 356–369.

——. 1987a. 'Making Women Visible in the Embryo Experimentation Debate.' In: *Bioethics* 1(2):179–188.

——. 1987b. 'Of women born, but for how long? The relationship of women to the new reproductive technologies and the issue of choice. In: *Made to Order*. Spallone and Steinberg (eds):67–83.

——. *Woman Herself. A Transdisciplinary Perspective on Women's Identity*. Oxford University Press, Melbourne.

Sattaur, Omar. 1984. 'New conception threatened by old morality'. In: *New Scientist* September 27th 1984: 13–14.

Scutt, Jocelynne (ed.) 1988. *The Baby Machine. Commercialisation of Motherhood*. McCulloch, Melbourne.

Singer, Peter and Deanne Wells. 1984. *The Reproductive Revolution. New Ways of Makinq Babies*. Oxford University Press, UK.

Sozialwissenschaftliche Forschung und Praxis fuer Frauen (Hrsg). 1986. *Frauen zwischen Auslese und Ausmerze. Beitraege zur feministischen Theorie und Praxis* Vol. 14, Cologne.

Spallone, Patricia. 1988. *Beyond Conception. The New Politics of Reproduction*. Macmillan, London.

—— and Steinberg, Deborah L. (eds). 1987. *Made to Order. The Myth of*

Reproductive and Genetic Progress. Pergamon Press, Oxford and New York.

Stanley, Fiona J. 1988. '*In vitro* fertilization — a gift for the infertile or a cycle of despair?' *Medical Journal of Australia* 148 (May 2):425–426.

Stanworth, Michelle (ed.). 1987. *Gender, Motherhood and Medicine*. Polity Press, Cambridge, UK.

Trounson, Alan. 1987. Future Directions of IVF. Presented at the Annual Meeting of the Licensing Executive Society, Sydney, March 1987.

Voluntary Licensing Authority for Human *In Vitro* Fertilisation and Embryology. 1987. Second Report April 1987, London.

Weikert, Aurelia, Riegler, Johanna and Trallori, Lisbeth N. (Hrsg). 1987. *Schoene Neue Maennerwelt. Beitraege zu Gen- und Fortpflanzungstechnologien*. Verlag fuer Gesellschaftskritik, Wien.

Winkler, Ute and Schönenberg, Traute. 1988. 'Options for Involuntarily Childless Women.' In: *Infertility. Women Speak Out About Their Experiences of Reproductive Medicine*, Klein (ed.):207–226.

Zipfel, Gaby (Hg). 1987. *Reproduktionsmedizin. Die Enteignung der weiblichen Natur*. Konkret Literatur Verlag, Hamburg.

★

JOURNAL

Reproductive and Genetic Engineering: Journal of International Feminist Analysis. Pergamon Press, New York and Oxford.

